Ophthalmology:

A Symptom-based Approach

Third edition

Ophthalmology:
A Symptom-based Approach

Third edition

Hector Bryson Chawla MBChB(St And)
DO(Lond) DRCOG(Lond) FRCS(Edin) FRCOphth
Consultant Ophthalmic Surgeon Royal Infirmary of Edinburgh
Examiner, Royal College of Surgeons, Edinburgh and the
Royal College of Ophthalmologists, London, UK

BUTTERWORTH
HEINEMANN

OXFORD   AUCKLAND   BOSTON   JOHANNESBURG   MELBOURNE   NEW DELHI

Butterworth-Heinemann
Linacre House, Jordan Hill, Oxford OX2 8DP
225 Wildwood Avenue, Woburn, MA 01801-2041
A division of Reed Educational and Professional Publishing Ltd

◭ A member of the Reed Elsevier plc group

First published as *Essential Ophthalmology* (CLMT) 1981
Revised for the Student Notes Series 1988
Second edition 1993
Reprinted 1994, 1997
Third edition 1999

British Library Cataloguing in Publication Data
A catalogue record for this book is available from the British Library

Library of Congress Cataloguing in Publication Data
A catalogue record for this book is available from the Library of Congress

ISBN 0 7506 3979 2

Composition by Scribe Design, Gillingham, Kent
Printed and bound in Italy

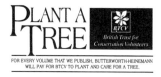

FOR EVERY VOLUME THAT WE PUBLISH, BUTTERWORTH-HEINEMANN
WILL PAY FOR BTCV TO PLANT AND CARE FOR A TREE.

Contents

Preface

The main obstacle to learning anything about the eye is ophthalmology itself. Its jargon obscures even the simplest idea and the quaintly named disorders are frequently taught as a mixture of pathology and therapeutics, with presenting features hidden somewhere in the middle. And at the beginning, a panorama of the ocular interior, caught in technicolour with the fundus camera, fosters the illusion that the same view will be caught with the direct ophthalmoscope.

The reality is, at best, little circles of red, usually out of focus. Yet these shadowy glimpses are generally regarded as a substitute for any attempt to assess ocular function and the whole subject has now become a collection of idealized fundal impressions that nobody ever sees.

This book tries to put things in order. Presenting features are placed at the beginning, because that is what patients present with. The limitations of the direct ophthalmoscope (the author does not have one) place it like the stethoscope, where it belongs, at the end of a ritual of examination that never changes.

Such is the way with the rest of medicine. If the ritual does not tell us what is wrong, it will certainly tell us what is not wrong, leaving us with a safe eye that will not go blind because we have missed something.

Acknowledgements

Acknowledgement is due to:

Ethicon Limited, PO Box 408, Bankhead Avenue, Edinburgh, Scotland EH11 4HE, Tel.: 0131 453 5555, Fax: 0131 453 6011 for their sponsorship of this book.

Stuart Gairns, who placed his photographic skills at my disposal.

Ian Lennox, whose crisp illustrations save paragraphs of print.

My wife Anna, for curbing my flights of fancy.

My daughter Louise, who modelled the examination sequences.

Sandra McDonagh, my secretary, who brought my scattered and often changing thoughts into coherent order.

1

The normal eye

In most textbooks of ophthalmology the initial impulse to simplicity quietly succumbs to the temptations of completeness. Any common link between the tissues of the eye and its host is lost in a recital of its unique behaviour. And the resultant miscellany of information, obscured by ophthalmobabble, is made finally incomprehensible by an explanatory section on optics.

This book regards the eye as just another part of the body that happens to contain some brain tissue and that happens to be partially transparent. Its structure can be likened to that of a hybrid drinking vessel – a brandy goblet with an eccentric stem and the lid of a German beer tankard.

Figure 1.1
The brandy goblet with lid. The rim of the lid marks the union between the anterior and posterior segments of the eye

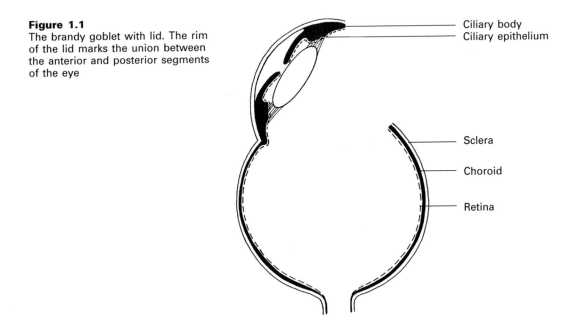

Ciliary body
Ciliary epithelium

Sclera

Choroid

Retina

The rim of the brandy goblet corresponds to:

- the insertion of the rectus muscles – external
- the ora serrata which marks the internal border between
  (a) the posterior limit of the ciliary body and
  (b) the anterior limit of the retina (ora serrata).

The retina can be compared to kitchen cellophane, lining the cavity of the goblet, attached at the rim and attached at the stem and potentially separable everywhere else. The cavity contains a structure like half-set clear jelly – the vitreous, also attached at the rim and attached at the stem.

The lid of the brandy goblet contains:

- the cornea
- the iris and ciliary body
- the lens.

The construction of the eye is therefore not as complicated as traditional teaching would have us believe and its capacity to transmit light is a key to understanding its behaviour. This transparency is dependent on a series of mechanisms that involve not only the external eye but most importantly the aqueous fluid. Although the eye is happiest when shut, the arrangement of tears, conjunctiva and eyelids does not exist simply to create comfort but rather to maintain the front of the cornea as an optical surface of quality.

Figure 1.2
The eye is happiest when shut. Comfort when open is maintained by the eyelids, which blink with the tear film across the cornea. The conjunctiva contributes lipids and mucus and mobility. The eye in the orbit is essentially a ball and socket joint

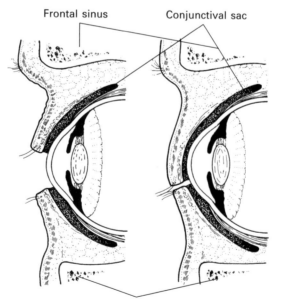

Frontal sinus   Conjunctival sac

Maxillary sinus

The tears and eyelids

Tears from the lacrimal gland, a suspension of mucus and lipid in salt solution, are continually blinked over the smooth surface of the cornea by the eyelids.

The cornea

- The entire structure is free of blood vessels, which, if present, would interfere with the passage of light.
- The cells in the body of the cornea (stroma) are arranged in a regular lattice pattern.
- The deep surface (endothelium) continually withdraws water from the cornea, keeping it in a state of partial hydration.

Figure 1.3
The corneal endothelium maintains corneal clarity by constant abstraction of water from the stroma

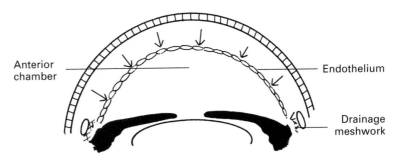

The lens

The regular avascular structure permits the free transmission of light.

The aqueous

The transparent structures – the cornea, the lens and the vitreous – in order to remain transparent, have to be nourished by a transparent blood substitute. This aqueous fluid arises from the ciliary epithelium. It percolates backwards through the vitreous, forwards through the pupil and fills the anterior chamber, out of which it drains through the trabecular meshwork, in the angle between the iris and the cornea.

The production and outflow of aqueous is continuous. It not only feeds the transparent tissues but maintains the shape and structure of the eye as well. Although it also differs from blood in that its circulation is not a fixed volume and that it does not clot, aqueous and blood have more things in common than not.

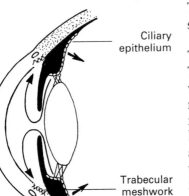

Figure 1.4
The ciliary body is the heart of the eye. Aqueous, produced by the ciliary epithelium, percolates into the vitreous, feeds the lens and passes through the pupil into the anterior chamber whence it departs via the trabecular meshwork

- The ciliary epithelium and the ciliary body are the heart of the eye.
- The aqueous plays the role of the blood.

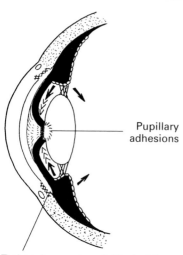

Trabecular meshwork blocked by forward iris

Figure 1.5
The aqueous flow obstructed by adhesions at the pupil. The iris bows forwards. The anterior chamber shallows. The intraocular pressure rises

Figure 1.6
A deep anterior chamber from the inside

- Without either there would be no eye and no vision.

DISTURBANCE OF THE AQUEOUS FLOW

Just as the pulse and blood pressure of the general circulation can be disturbed by a range of pathological influences, so can the pressure of the eye.

Every time something happens to an eye, we must presume some disturbance to the passage of aqueous until we prove there be none.

Blockage of aqueous on its journey from the ciliary body, through the pupil to the drainage angle will result in a raised intraocular pressure. When the pressure of the eyeball rises above the pressure of blood feeding the optic nerve, two things happen.

- Defects develop within the field of vision.
- The optic nerve begins to atrophy in a cupped fashion.

These three features then

- raised intraocular pressure
- field defect
- optic nerve head cupping

are the marks of **glaucoma** – the pathological process.

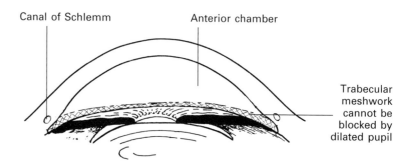

The intraocular pressure, like the blood pressure, almost always rises without symptoms. Measuring the blood pressure is a routine check in general medicine. So is measurement of the intraocular pressure in ophthalmology.
This is the first key.

THE EYE IS A ONE-RESPONSE ORGAN

Each part of the eye tends to behave in the same way,

whatever pathological process may strike. The well-known catalogue of insult

- congenital
- hereditary
- traumatic
- inflammatory
- neoplastic
- toxic
- degenerative
- vascular
- metabolic etc.

can affect the eye just as they can affect everything else.

Should any one of these diverse influences involve the lens, the lens will have one solitary response: it will develop a cataract (though to be pedantically accurate, trauma can lead to dislocation as well).

When we then consider the diagnosis of conditions that appear to multiply beyond reason, we should not ask the question – What pathological process is affecting the eye? Rather we should ask, *What part of the eye is affected?*

This is the second key

Thus, the two key questions are:

- Is the intraocular pressure raised?
- Which part of the eye is affected? (It is a one-response organ.)

THE NORMAL EYE

Vision

The whole point of the eye is to see, but what is not generally recognized is that vision is not all of a piece and breaks up into two distinct parts – central and field. Although they are both served by the same retina they are quite separate in position and quite different in function.

Whilst it is customary to liken the eye to a wide-angled camera, it has to be said that the eye came first and there are major dissimilarities. The 'retina' of the camera – the film – is flat; the retina of the eye on the other hand takes on the concave shape of the vitreal cavity. There are other differences: the camera does not discriminate what it records; detail is equal throughout. The eye does discriminate; it picks out one object to fix on with its central vision which, playing over an observed scene, creates the impression that all aspects of the scene are perceived in the same detail at the same time. They are not. It is an illusion, created because the eye is moving, not fixed and staring. When the eye stares at one object, other objects, remote from the point of fixation, are not made out in detail. It is for this reason that holiday snapshots are so terribly disappointing.

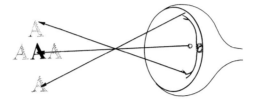

Figure 1.7
Foveal detail may appear to dominate vision, but objects in the field, like brush strokes on a canvas, form a very essential background against which to appreciate macular detail. The macula, constantly scanning, creates the illusion that all vision is detailed. It is for this reason that attempts to capture landscapes with a camera are almost always disappointing

Central vision

The visual axis runs from the macula through the pupil to whatever has been selected for detailed observation. The central retina measures about 1.5 mm – the same size as the optic nerve. The macula at its centre is tiny – 0.5 mm and the central area of that – the fovea – for even greater detail, is even smaller still. Upon this area depends colour sense and that faculty for distinguishing between almost similar details which is the very essence of central visual acuity.

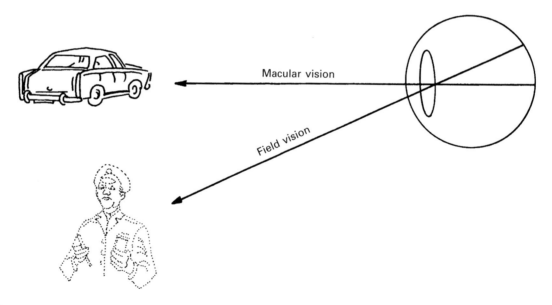

Macular vision

Field vision

Figure 1.8
The car is seen sharply. The warden's pleasure is but an impression until the macula fixes on his triumph

Field vision

Most patients and a few doctors are not aware of the existence of the visual field. It is none the less the greater part of vision. Not concerned with detail or the recognition of colour, however, it gives critical awareness of position in space and allows the eye to adapt to darkness.

Normal sight (central vision)

Such an eye brings parallel rays of light to focus from infinity (6+ metres) without effort. Normal distance acuity is recorded as 6/6 (20/20 feet). The upper figure is the distance at which the test is carried out – 6 metres. The lower figure is the distance at which letter size ought to be seen – 6 metres. 6/12 means that the eye in question can only make out at 6 metres a letter size that it ought to make out at 12 metres.

Figure 1.9
The normal-sighted eye discerns detail in distance without effort. The convexity of the lens, increased by the ciliary muscle, allows the same for near until advancing age around the mid-forties stops the lens from responding

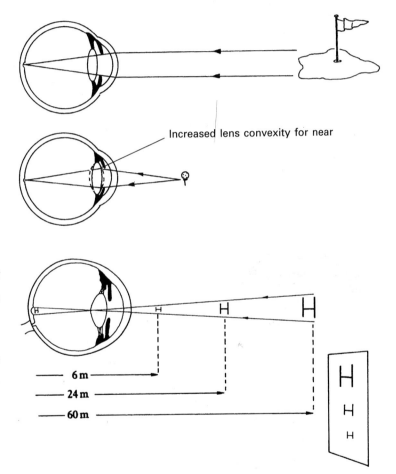

Increased lens convexity for near

Figure 1.10
The Snellen chart. The 6 metre letter at 6 metres and the 60 metre letter at 60 metres appear the same to the eye, because they bend light to the same degree. Larger letters, closer to the eye, are perceived as large because the closer they are to the eye, the more they bend the light. A simple magnifying glass allows objects to be seen nearer to the eye than the eye can normally manage on its own. It is therefore useless in extreme myopes who cannot bring things any closer without the threat of a penetrating injury

6 m
24 m
60 m

Near vision

The normal eye can shift its focus from infinity to near. Just how near diminishes with age, but most children with chastening skill can discern detail at a couple of inches from the eye. The muscular part of the ciliary body contracts. The elastic tension on the lens capsule steepens its surface into a greater convexity. The lens becomes more powerful and shortens its focal length.

Figure 1.11
Near vision: contraction of the ciliary body increases the lens convexity

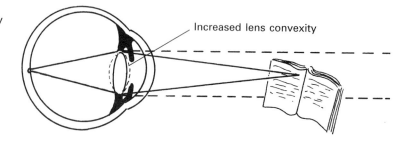

Increased lens convexity

As the years go by, the hardening lens is indifferent to the contraction of the ciliary muscle and, by the mid-forties, most people find that the arms are now too short for comfortable reading. Such is the explanation of presbyopia. This rigidity of focus, is a quality that might describe certain types of clergymen and it is not without irony that the word presbyterian shares the same derivation.

Figure 1.12
Presbyopia: the denied evidence of passing time. The printer's ink is not what it used to be in the good old days and the arms are becoming too short

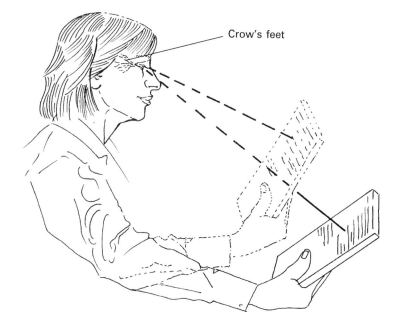

Crow's feet

ERRORS OF REFRACTION

Long sight (hypermetropia)
The focal length of this eye is longer than the eye itself. The focal point would therefore lie behind the retina, were light

able to pass through to reach it. In order to focus on the macula, the ciliary muscle has to contract as for reading and uses up its whole range of focus for near to see in the distance.

Figure 1.13
The long-sighted eye cannot see detail in the distance without effort and has to use up its near focus to do so. Before the mid-forties, a convex lens for distance allows the natural range of focus to operate. After that age presbyopia strikes again as well

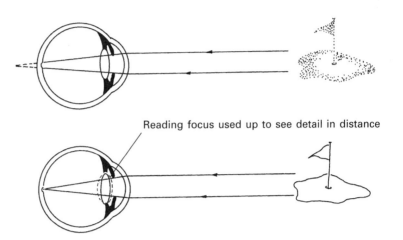

Reading focus used up to see detail in distance

Such eyes may find near focusing impossible. Without glasses, a 30-year-old with long sight could be as helpless for near as would a 50-year-old presbyope.

For the long-sighted 30-year-old, a convex lens compensates for the distance defect, releasing the normal extent of focus of that age group, to allow clear vision at the common reading distance.

Short sight

The focal length of such an eye is too short for the eyeball. Parallel rays from distant objects, do not reach the macula. Such objects are blurred. They become clearer the nearer

Figure 1.14
The short-sighted eye cannot make out detail in the distance with or without effort on the part of the ciliary muscle. Effort by the eyelids, on the other hand, can screw them into a slit, simulating the effect of a pinhole at the price of crows' feet trampling all over the skin where they are most visible

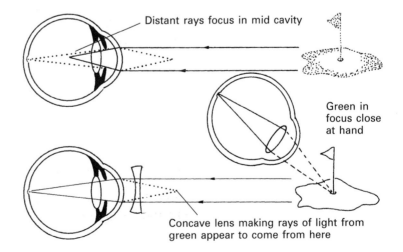

Distant rays focus in mid cavity

Green in focus close at hand

Concave lens making rays of light from green appear to come from here

they approach the eye because the now divergent rays of light, like a speeding car, take longer to come to a halt at their point of focus.

Astigmatism

In simple long sight and short sight the optical mechanisms are round and bring rays of light to a point focus on the macula with a round correction. Sometimes however, these mechanisms are not round, but oval and focus more in one meridian than in another.

Figure 1.15
Astigmatism: a point focus is impossible because the eye is not equal in all meridians. This eye is normal-sighted in the vertical meridian but short-sighted in the horizontal meridian. The focus is oval and all is blurred

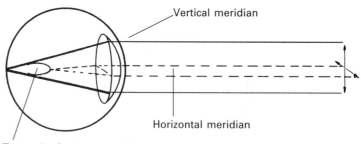

Vertical meridian

Horizontal meridian

Two point foci separated by an oval

Instead of bringing rays of light to a point they bring them to an oval, horizontally elongated in proportion to the degree of astigmatism. The answer, therefore, is an oval lens which focuses in one meridian only, to make the eye effectively an optical sphere once more.

Figure 1.16
The left homonymous field. The right half of the retina of each eye serves the left visual field. It is for this reason that vision in one eye may be lost in the comforting misbelief that both eyes are functioning properly

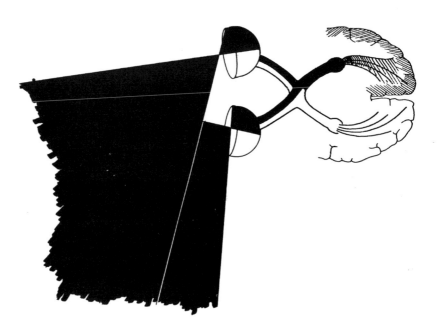

Field vision

The right and left visual pathway each carry half the impulses from each retina to the occipital cortex. Beyond the chiasma for example the left optic tract and radiation transmit impulses from corresponding points in the left half of the left retina and the left half of the right retina. Such is the explanation of field loss on one side of the body (homonymous hemianopia) when the optic radiation in the opposite side of the brain are damaged.

The monocular field of each eye arranges itself naturally around the point of fixation of each eye. Textbooks illustrate this monocular field as a flat pear when it is in fact in three dimensions, like the cavity of half an avocado, with the contents removed. With both eyes open, the mirror image half-pear skins fuse together into one large binocular field.

Figure 1.17
Field of vision. That of each eye extends in the shape of an empty avocado pear skin – upwards, forwards, downwards and to the sides. Normal binocular vision fuses these monocular fields into one three-dimensional sense of depth. A crescent of vision along the temporal boundary of each field belongs to that eye alone

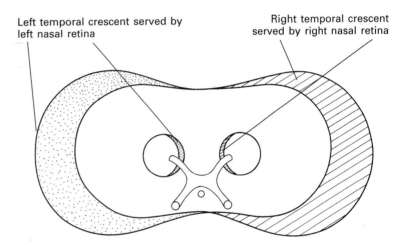

Left temporal crescent served by left nasal retina

Right temporal crescent served by right nasal retina

A monocular crescent makes up the temporal extremity on each side.

This non-macular vision spreads beyond 180 degrees on the temporal side and angles forwards across the nose (although not because of the nose) on the nasal side. It tends to be forgotten that it spreads also upwards and downwards and may be likened to a spray of buckshot from an eccentric blunderbuss.

2

A common process at work in a special organ

Every specialty nurses the firm belief that it is unique – yet there are more similarities than otherwise. A system goes wrong. Patients complain. Doctors interfere, and the only difference is where it all happens. There is actually only a limited range of things that can go wrong. It is regional variations that make them seem inexhaustible.

The fundamental processes in pathology are but few and nothing could be more fundamental than inflammation. Whatever its site, it is characterized by:

- redness – rubor
- heat – calor
- pain – dolor
- swelling – tumor
- loss of function – since the Romans and indeed the Victorians never recognized any such thing in themselves, no Latin tag ever came into popular use.

Figure 2.1
Acute iritis

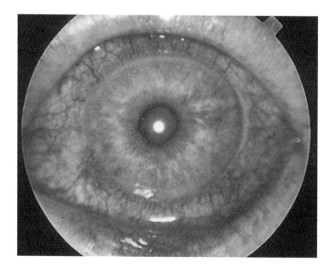

The intention of this chapter is to demonstrate, using inflammation of the iris as a model, how symptoms and signs can be worked out on a reasoned basis and how on the same reasoned basis a system of management can be evolved, founded on certainty rather than hope.

The iris is the anterior part of that complex known as the uveal tract. The origins of iris inflammation differ in no way from the origins of such inflammation anywhere else.

Whatever its site, an acute inflammatory attack can generally do one of four things. It may:

- Resolve without damage to special tissue.
- Retreat after special tissue has been replaced with functionless fibrous tissue.
- Spread to an adjacent structure.
- Continue to smoulder as a chronic disease process.

None of this information can be regarded as either novel or obscure.

IN THE EYE

Acute phase

Figure 2.2
Ciliary injection: the major sign of a serious red eye. The whole ciliary body is inflamed but only the part adjacent to the corneo-scleral limbus is visible. The spastic pupil suggests inflammation of the iris

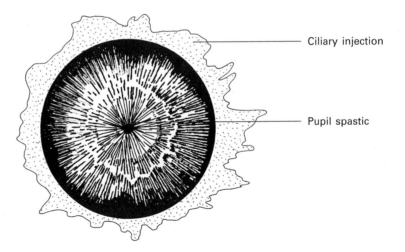

Ciliary injection

Pupil spastic

- Blood vessels at the margin of the cornea become inflamed.
- The iris swells and releases exudate into the anterior chamber.
- The iris sphincter muscle goes into spasm, painfully constricting the pupil.
- Inflammatory debris, dancing about in the visual field will be described as floaters.

Figure 2.3
Adhesions between the iris and the lens block the flow of aqueous in its passage to the anterior chamber. The pupil is not only spastic but stuck down in an irregular fashion

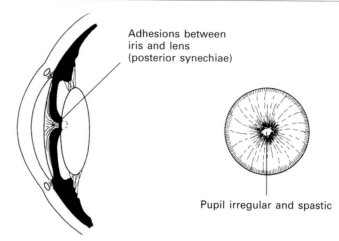

Adhesions between iris and lens (posterior synechiae)

Pupil irregular and spastic

It can also silt up the drainage angle, blocking the flow of aqueous.

Chronic phase

- The proceeding inflammation may produce adhesions (synechiae) between adjacent structures – most usually the iris and the lens.
- The toxic aqueous can poison the lens into a cataract.

Figure 2.4
The consequence of iris lens adhesions. The obstructed aqueous builds up behind the pupil, pushing the iris forward into the anterior chamber – iris bombeé, another cause of raised intraocular pressure

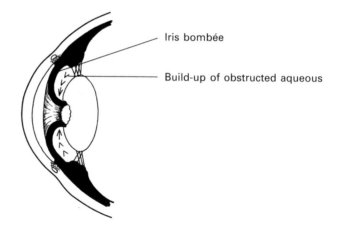

Iris bombée

Build-up of obstructed aqueous

None of the preceding information is unpredictable and should serve to remind us that pathological conditions, like deciduous leaves, bud, spread and wither.

HOW THE EYE IS DISTURBED

- Vision is usually affected one way or another.
- Inflammation develops around the corneal margin.

Figure 2.5
The lens is the hub of the ciliary wheel: the pars plana of the ciliary body forms the spokes. The posterior edge of the pars plana merges with the anterior edge of the retina (ora serrata)

Rectus insertions mark border between pars plana and retina

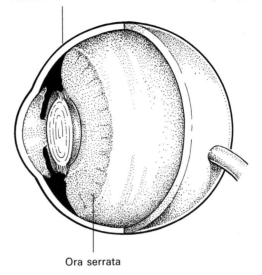

Ora serrata

- Inflammatory debris in the drainage angle will block the aqueous flow and the intraocular pressure will rise.
- Inflammatory debris on the deep surface of the cornea impairs the endothelial suction pump, hydrating and clouding the stroma and epithelium.
- Adhesions developing between the iris and the lens may block the flow of aqueous. The iris ballooning forwards is given the name iris bombeé. Whatever the fanciful title, the intraocular pressure will rise.
- The lens, bathed by aqueous, poisoned by inflammation and possibly by therapeutic corticosteroids as well, responds in the only way it can by losing its transparency – by any other name, a cataract.

If the condition fails to resolve or does not respond to treatment or continues to grumble, the chronic process will eventually destroy the ciliary body. The aqueous flow diminishes and the eyeball will shrink.

All the preceding effects are predictable from:

- The application of general principles to an organ which happens to be special.
- Remembering to consider that something is likely to have happened to the aqueous circulation.

MANAGEMENT

The scheme of management of any condition does not differ whatever organ is involved. It can be divided into:

- *short term medical*
- *short term surgical*
- *long term medical*
- *long term surgical*.

Into this frame work can be slotted those principles common to all branches of medicine, that:

- The exciting cause be removed – if possible.
- If the cause be not known, then the destructive processes be curbed – if possible.
- Complications be anticipated (it should be remembered that remedies frequently have complications also).
- Pain be relieved.
- Function be restored.

Short term medical

As the cause of the inflammation is not usually known, we have to move straight on to principle 2 and curb the inflammatory process with topical corticosteroids. The frequency of dosage must be tailored to the severity of the condition. Four times a day to the eye has acquired an almost scriptural sanctity, but in many cases every hour would be more appropriate.

We should mention at this point that long term use of corticosteroids may be as toxic to the eye as the disease itself:

- It may upset the aqueous balance which in turn will upset the lens which in turn will respond in the only way it can, with a cataract.
- It may also raise the intraocular pressure.

Figure 2.6
Pupil partially dilated by mydriatics and partially stuck down by adhesions between the iris and the lens

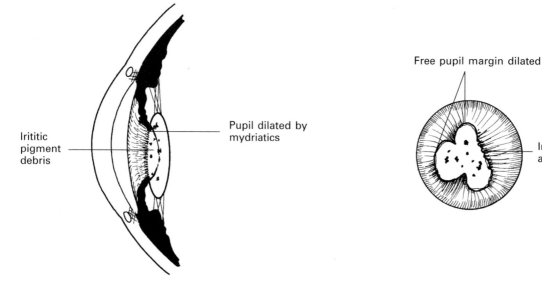

Irititic pigment debris

Pupil dilated by mydriatics

Free pupil margin dilated

Iris lens adhesions

Iris lens adhesions can more easily block the entire circumference of a small pupil than of a large pupil. The pupil must therefore be dilated with some suitable agent. Atropine drops have a long pedigree and are long acting. The drug acquires the name of belladonna from the custom of Roman ladies of fashion. They applied a decoction of atropine to turn their eyes into black pools of seduction, charming to a succession of misshapen consorts whose own shortcomings would be less obvious to eyes that could not see them clearly.

If the flow of aqueous has been obstructed, then the raised pressure has to be reduced. This can be done in two ways:

- The inflow of aqueous can be reduced.
- The outflow of aqueous can be increased.

Acetazolamide, a carbonic anhydrase inhibitor, reduces the production of aqueous. A whole range of anti-pressure drops now exists but the one not to use is pilocarpine because constriction of the pupil is the last thing we want in iritis.

In the short term we are not generally concerned with perfect function but we must remember that the eye will want to see again later. Analgesics possibly, an assurance certainly will be required because all people have an unspoken terror of going blind.

Long term management
The ongoing complications of smouldering chronic iritis require definitive attention. If the pressure remains high, it will call for

- continued topical medication. If this fails, then
- surgery may bypass the obstructions:
  (a) blockage at the pupil can be relieved by a hole cut in the iris (iridectomy) to allow the aqueous to drain from the posterior chamber into the anterior chamber and out – *provided the drainage meshwork is intact.*
  (b) If the drainage meshwork is not intact then an external drain (trabeculectomy) will allow the aqueous fluid to continue its passage from the anterior chamber, out of the eye.
  (c) Should the lens have succumbed either to the disease or the treatment, then cataract extraction is the only way of allowing light back into the eye again. Such an extra extraction removes a vital element in the ocular focus but to replace it with a lens implant in the presence of an uncontained iritis may elevate the process to even greater heights of activity.

Figure 2.7
Pupil block relieved by peripheral
iridectomy

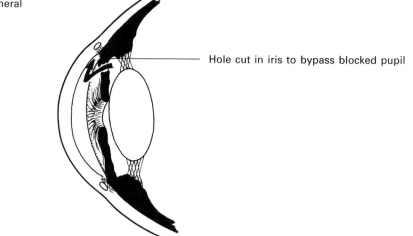

Hole cut in iris to bypass blocked pupil

Figure 2.8
Trabeculectomy: external drainage
operation to relieve raised
intraocular pressure. The aqueous
now passes from the anterior
chamber into the subconjunctival
space

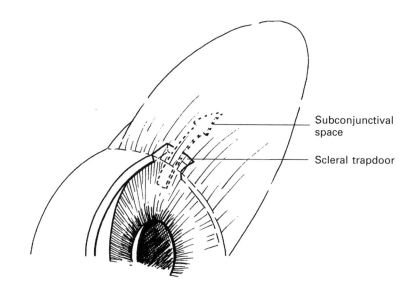

Subconjunctival
space

Scleral trapdoor

3

What patients complain about

As every examination candidate says,

'I would take a good history'

thus prompting the question

'What other sort of history would you take?'

The principles of history-taking, well established in general medicine, are no different in ophthalmology. However, one question above all will separate serious ocular complaints from all the rest.
'Is the vision affected?'

WHAT PATIENTS COMPLAIN OF

There are five main symptoms:

- alteration in appearance
- pain
- watering (with or without discharge)
- alteration in vision
- double vision.

Only the last two are strictly ocular. Normal appearances are well enough known for any variation to be obvious. Pain can occur anywhere, while the lacrimal apparatus is really a lubricating gland and drainage system that happen to lie beside the eye.

Almost more important is none of these five, but the following.

WHAT PATIENTS DO NOT COMPLAIN ABOUT

Elevation of intraocular pressure
A rising intraocular pressure is almost always without symptoms. This rule is broken only when the rise is rapid,

Figure 3.1
Proptosis: orbital neoplasm

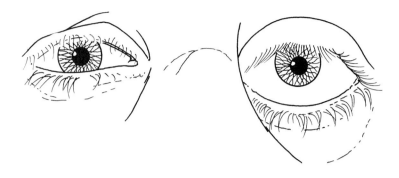

as in acute angle closure where the anterior chamber is too shallow for the pupil to dilate safely.

Loss of visual field

Since most people are unaware that there is such a thing, it is not surprising that much of it can be lost without their being aware of that either. We might ask

'Why is the field so important if it can be lost so casually?'

It is so, because most of the visual field is binocular and since both eyes are usually open at the same time, the field of one can slip away unnoticed.

When we are pursuing symptoms that people complain of we must always pursue the two features they do not complain of and ask ourselves:

- Has something happened to the intraocular pressure?
- Has something happened to the visual field?

4

The ophthalmic ritual

Ophthalmic clinical signs are as limitless and sometimes as obscure as the milky way date from the days when someone's triad or someone else's tetrad were a substitute for an explanation. They are not however a substitute for a system of examination. In ophthalmology this system is based on seven simple observations and an occasional eighth. Observations are made and signs are found and may expand at a clinician's fancy but the observations never change in kind or number, whatever the complaint and whatever the condition.

The first three involve vision:

- central for distance
- central for near
- field.

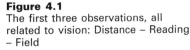

Figure 4.1
The first three observations, all related to vision: Distance – Reading – Field

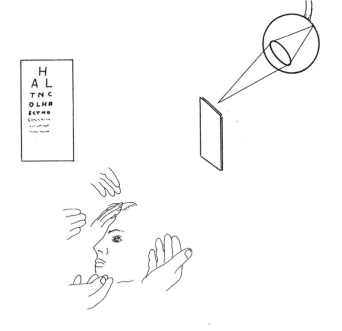

The second three involve the essential external eye:

- the state of the cornea
- the state of the pupil
- the depth of the anterior chamber.

Figure 4.2
The second three observations, all related to the external eye: – Cornea – Pupil – Anterior chamber

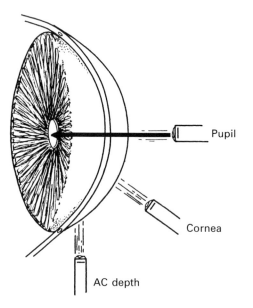

Next is the search for the asymptomatic sign:

7   the intraocular pressure (measured with the fingers).

Now and only now do we consider:

8   the direct ophthalmoscope, an instrument of such limitation that many ophthalmologists use something else.

Like the stethoscope, the direct ophthalmoscope should be used only to confirm what we expect to find. At best it allows a view of the posterior pole of the eyeball in little circular segments. In practice, this means the optic nerve head, the adjacent vessels and the macula.

To attempt this, with the pupil undilated, in a sunlit ward, with a waning battery and no idea of how the eye performs, is a feat much prized by physicians and not rated by ophthalmologists. The same physician would not apply a stethoscope without checking that the patient is at least breathing ...

The answer to their favourite question

'What do you make of that fundus?'

has to be

'Nothing until I have gone through the ritual of ophthalmic observations and even after that, nothing until the pupil has been dilated.'

The safe eye

A safe eye is one that will not go blind because we have missed something.

If we cannot find out what is wrong every time, *at least we know what is not wrong* – that the visual field is intact and the intraocular pressure normal; in other words, that the patient will be safe, provided no new symptoms arise.

ASSESSMENT OF VISION

Central vision

Central vision fails for two reasons:

- a refractive error (the need for spectacles)
- something is interfering with macular function (not necessarily the macula itself).

The Snellen chart (distance vision)

Starting with a letter that should be seen by the healthy eye at 60 metres, the Snellen chart reduces the letters step by step until they are of size that should be seen at 6 metres – the distance at which the test is carried out.

It goes without saying that the faded heirlooms found in every medical ward, where the letters, off grey, merge into a background, off white, are not exactly what Snellen had in mind.

Central vision for distance should be checked one eye at a time. A normal eye will, at 6 metres, see a letter size which ought to be seen at 6 metres and the vision recorded as 6/6 (20/20 feet). If the patient can only see a letter size at 6 metres which ought to be seen at 12 metres then the vision will be recorded as 6/12 and, it should be remembered, outside the car driving standard.

Refractive error

If the central vision for distance does not come up to standard then we have to know if such a spectacle correction might be necessary.

The pinhole disc

Eyes with spectacle errors and no spectacles bend rays of light to a focal point, but one not on the macula. In all optical systems, however, there is one central ray not deviated because there is nothing to deviate it and so it must

Figure 4.3
Every bundle of rays from every
point is reduced to one ray and each
of them is in focus. If central vision
improves with a pinhole, it can
improve with glasses

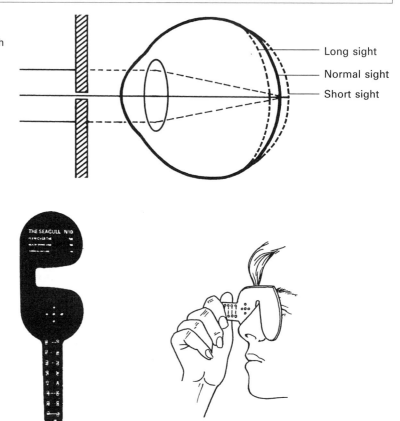

Long sight

Normal sight

Short sight

reach the macula no matter what the refractive error –
provided the effect of that error can be nullified.

The pinhole eliminates all other rays, allowing only the
central ray to pass on its own. If the macula has the potential to see, the pinhole disc will prove it. Acuity worsening
with a pinhole suggests an opacity on the axial line.

Near vision

Failure to see the smallest print without correction may
simply mean that reading spectacles are required, and in
most people they are – after the age of 40.

The pinhole disc applies equally for near as well as it does
for distance.

NB: It is not always necessary to test for both distance
and near.

- Good distance acuity makes near measurement superfluous.
- Poor distance acuity, however, can occur in an eye with
reasonable macular function but a severe refractive
error.

In these circumstances, good near acuity indicates a functioning macula.

Vision not recordable with figures
If the vision is not good enough to be granted numbers, we record it in descending order of quality as:

- counting fingers (CF)
- hand movements (HM)
- perception of light (PL).

Field of vision
In general terms, lesions anterior to the chiasma affect one eye only. Lesions at the chiasma produce temporal defects in both fields. Lesions behind the chiasma pick up the temporal fibres from one eye and the nasal fibres from its fellow and must produce a corresponding field defect in each eye (homonymous) – temporal for one and nasal for the other.

There are two aspects to the visual field:

- The outer contour (important for this examination sequence).
- The inner quality.

The outer contour
This is the only bit of the field that we should be seriously concerned with. In its basic simplicity it is most informative and a routine part of the cranial nerve examination. Recurrent attempts to turn it into something it is not – pins with coloured heads, finger counting and the like, masquerading

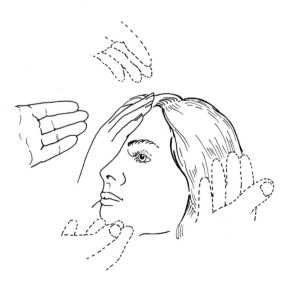

Figure 4.4
The outer limits of the visual field can be picked up with hand movements

as an assessment of inner quality – merely make likely that whatever we are looking for will not be found.

The outer contour can be picked up very easily one eye at a time, by asking if the fingers can be seen moving:

- 5 cm from the lateral orbital margin
- 5 cm in front of the fellow eye
- 5 cm from the chin
- 5 cm from the junction of the forehead with the scalp.

There is a firm if somewhat misguided belief that the examiner should carry out the test with one eye shut as well. This alleged confrontation of similar fields, with the hand moving half way between the patient and the examiner, far from comparing like with like, actually loses some 30 degrees of the temporal field of both examiner and patient. Each could have an enlarging pituitary and not know it. If someone came to us complaining of a sore left foot, the equivalent response would be for us to take off our right shoe.

Inner quality
Any gap within the field – a scotoma – can only be picked up:

- with uniform small targets
- against a uniform background
- with uniform illumination
- by people who do it often.

Area of visual field going
When side vision is faltering, an object large enough, in illumination bright enough, may be picked up, or when an

Figure 4.5
Relative field defect: the smaller monkey is not seen, the larger one is. If the illumination is increased the smaller one may be seen also

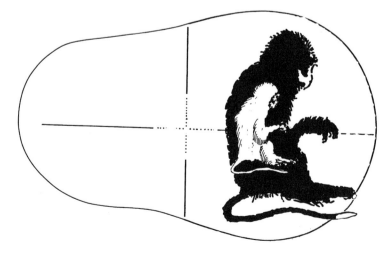

object smaller in illumination dimmer, may not. The defect is called relative. It is as though a baboon might be glimpsed to the side at noon and also at dusk whilst a monkey might be visible only at noon and maybe not even then.

Area of visual field gone

When the field loss is unambiguous, an object, no matter how large in illumination, no matter how bright, will not be visible. The defect is then described as absolute and in these circumstances, not even a gorilla would be picked up in the noon-day sun in the affected field although its very size might bring some of it into view in the centre.

Figure 4.6
Absolute field defect: the gorilla, being so big, spills into both sides of the visual field but is not seen on the right, no matter what the illumination. In the left field where it is visible, the part fixed on by the macula is seen in detail

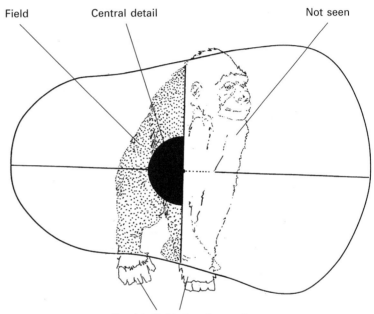

Field   Central detail   Not seen

Outside field, therefore not seen

Static perimetry

Automated field analysers are very popular today. They are unfortunately misnamed; they are not analysers but presenters. It is we who have to analyse, with increasing difficulty as their presentation becomes more and more complex.

Damato field test

Of recent invention, this ingenious contrivance utilizes what patients want to do most – use their central fixation and move their eyes. All other tests demand that the eyes remain still.

When the other eye is covered the patient is asked to follow the numbers from 1 to 26. This has the effect of running the central black dot on the chart over the visual

Figure 4.7
The Damato test allows the eye to move to areas of the field most at risk from raised pressure over a fixed point. Other tests require that the eyes do what they find most difficult – to fix on a point whilst something else moves in the field

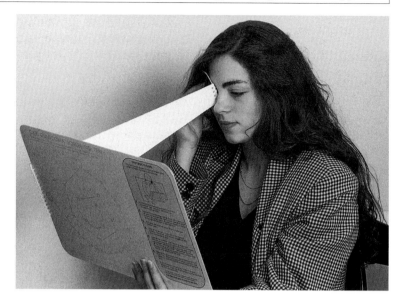

field within the margins of the cone where the scotomata of glaucoma are known to develop. If the black dot is visible at all times, there is no glaucoma loss.

Inattention

Patients with lesions of the parietal lobe may have deficiency in perception without actual loss of perception. When both the temporal and nasal field are tested at the same time, that field which corresponds to the damaged parietal lobe will give the impression of extinction. If each quadrant is tested separately then the danger of recording a defect that does not exist will be eliminated.

Figure 4.8
A dense cataract might reduce the field vision to below hand movements. It would have to be exceedingly dense to bring it below the level of light perception

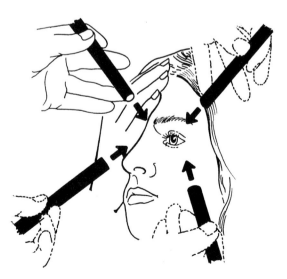

Light projection
When vision is reduced to perception of light, the capacity to point to light in different quadrants gives some clue about the field of vision.

THREE ESSENTIAL SIGNS IN THE ANTERIOR SEGMENT

These are the observation, palpation and percussion triad of the eye and *they must be carried out every time:*

*   The state of the cornea.
*   The state of the pupil.
*   The depth of the anterior chamber.

The state of the cornea
The cornea normally glistens and sparkles. Breaches in the corneal epithelium will be apparent in the light of a torch as a certain roughness. Areas deficient of epithelium will stain green with sodium fluorescein.

Figure 4.9
Applying fluorescein

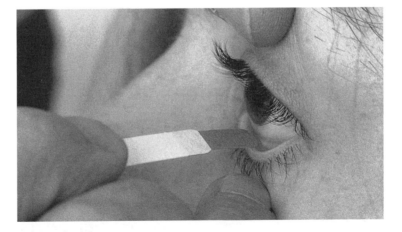

Figure 4.10
Corneal abrasion. The area of absent epithelium stains green with fluorescein

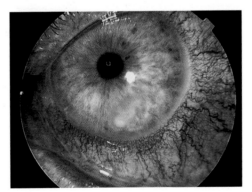

Figure 4.11
Superficial punctate keratitis:
multiple corneal erosions, the one
result of several causes – ultraviolet
light, tear deficiency, chemical
irritation

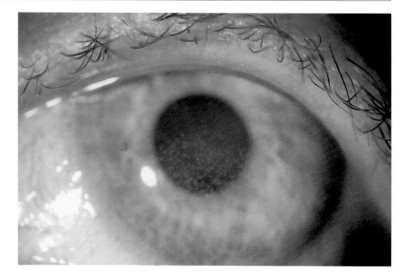

The state of the pupil

The pupil is that hole in the centre of the iris which changes size in response to:

- the level of light
- accommodation
- sympathetic activity
- certain drugs.

The stronger muscle, the sphincter, makes it contract. The weaker, the dilator, does the reverse.

The pupil regulates the amount of light entering the eye. There are two distinct reflex pathways:

- the response to light
- the response to near focus (accommodation).

The former is by far the more important.

The light reflex

All reflexes have an inflow and an outflow pathway and require a stimulus. The stimulus is light. Impulses travel by one or other optic nerve to the level of the mid-brain. From there they pass to both third nerve nucleii and via the ciliary ganglions to both pupils.

The test

The pupil confronted with a bright light constricts briskly and remains constricted. It tends to break free from this constriction (relative afferent pupillary defect) if any defect exists along the inflow pathway, e.g. optic neuritis. Such is

Figure 4.12
Normal pupils: both will constrict
(direct and consensual reflexes)
when either one is exposed to a
bright light

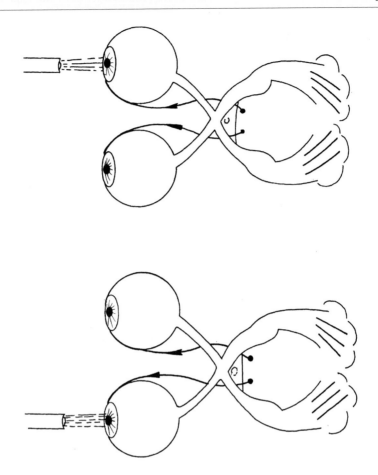

the essence of testing the pupil reflexes and any sophistication, as described under the separate section on pupils,
merely adds an extra layer of subtlety under the name of
the swinging light test.

Figure 4.13
Left inflow defect: illumination of
right eye – both pupils constrict;
illumination of left eye – neither
pupil constricts

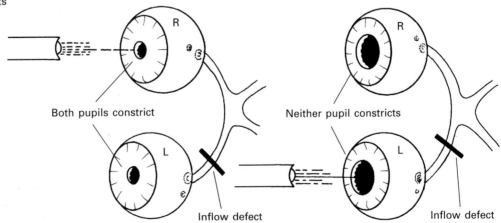

Both pupils constrict

Inflow defect

Neither pupil constricts

Inflow defect

Inflow defect
Such is the name we give to a dysfunction of the inflow pathway. As just described, it reduces or eliminates constriction of the pupil on:

- the affected side (direct reflex)
- the opposite side (consensual reflex).

Outflow defect
Dysfunction at any point along the third nerve to the pupil reduces or eliminates constriction on the affected side no matter which eye is illuminated.

Figure 4.14
Right outflow defect: illumination of right pupil – direct reflex absent, consensual reflex present; illumination of left pupil – direct reflex present, consensual reflex absent

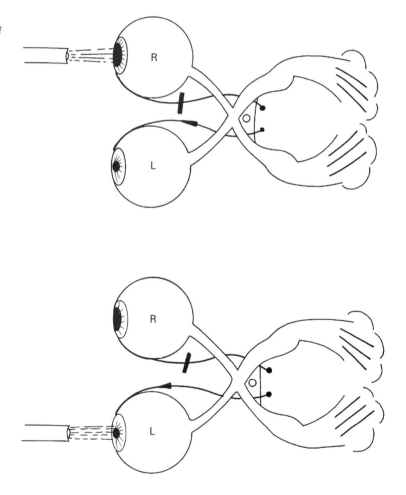

The accommodation reflex
Presentation of small print or of any other object of interest, particularly if the eye can focus, brings about constriction of the pupil.

Depth of the anterior chamber – the eclipse test

The anterior chamber is that space between the iris and the cornea. If it is deep the iris is gently convex. If it is shallow the iris is grossly convex – almost like a hillock with the pupil at its summit and one slope hidden from the other. This concealment, more pronounced as the anterior chamber becomes more shallow, is the basis of the eclipse test. It will indicate:

- when it is safe to dilate the pupil (it usually is)
- when it is not safe to dilate the pupil.

Of all the preventable conditions this must be one of the most preventable, yet whilst much time and effort are spent in the search for diagnostic trivia, the shallow anterior chambers of eyes, predictably prey to acute angle closure, are quietly ignored.

Figure 4.15
Using the ophthalmoscope as a torch to determine the depth of the anterior chamber – the eclipse test

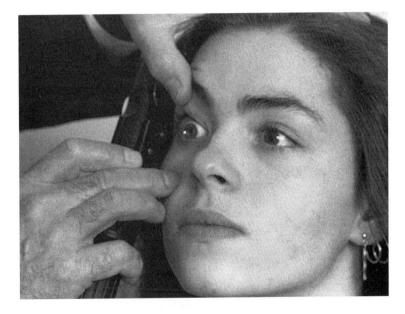

Figure 4.16
Eclipse test positive. The iris in a shallow anterior chamber is like a hillock with the pupil at its summit. Light falls on one side but the other is in shadow. Angle closure is possible when the pupil is dilated

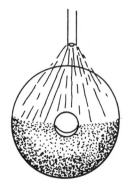

The test

A light directed from the margin of the cornea across the iris plane will illuminate as much of the anterior chamber as its depth allows.

- In a deep anterior chamber the entire iris will be suffused with light.
- In a shallow anterior chamber, only the half adjacent to the light will be illuminated:
  the remote half is in shadow
  the light is eclipsed.

Figure 4.17
Eclipse test negative. The anterior chamber is deep. The iris, more a plain than a hillock, is uniformly illuminated. The pupil may be dilated with impunity

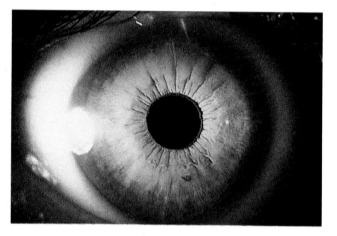

Figure 4.18
Eclipse test positive. The iris surface remote from the beam is in shadow. Angle closure is possible. Until something happens, this is not a disease but a shape

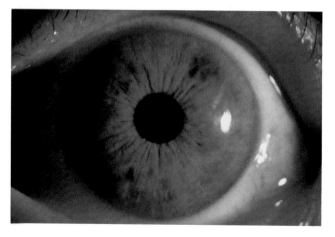

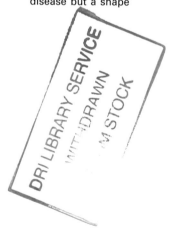

THE INTRAOCULAR PRESSURE

Digital tonometry

Through the eyelid above the tarsal plate we palpate the eye as we would a boil. The eye should look down, for the lid is at its thinnest just under the upper outer angle of the orbit. Both hands are stabilized by leaning on the patient's forehead with the sides of the ring fingers and pinkies. The middle or index fingers are thus released for palpation.

Figure 4.19
Not everyone has access to or the skill with a tonometer. The pinkie and ring fingers lean on the forehead, whilst the index or middle fingers are held firmly together, pulp to nail and firmly on the eye above the lateral end of the tarsal plate. A slight movement of one finger, sets up a shimmer of fluctuation sensed by the other finger

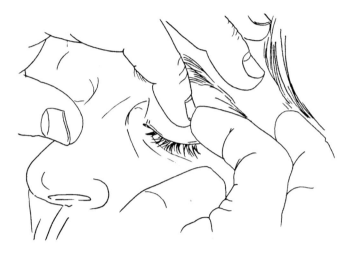

The palpating fingers brush together pulp to nail. They must maintain contact with each other and with the globe. One finger is active. One is passive. The mobile finger presses gently on the eye with a tiny alternating action, whilst the static finger senses the thrill of fluctuation. The softer the eye, the greater the fluctuation. And if doubt can ever bring comfort, the only certainty about a pressure palpated incorrectly is that it will feel high rather than low. To be wrong in this way is not a catastrophe.

OPHTHALMOSCOPY: THE EIGHTH OBSERVATION

As with the stethoscope, which deals in muffled murmurs, the ophthalmoscope deals in fleeting glimpses.

The instrument requires to correct refractive errors in:

- the observer
- the observed.

Such correction is achieved by rotating the disc of focus:

- anti-clockwise for short sight
- clockwise for long sight.

With the leading hand placed on the patient's forehead, right hand right eye, left hand left eye, the instrument is directed from the temporal side as if towards the pituitary

Figure 4.20
Examining the fundus – preferably
through the dilated pupil

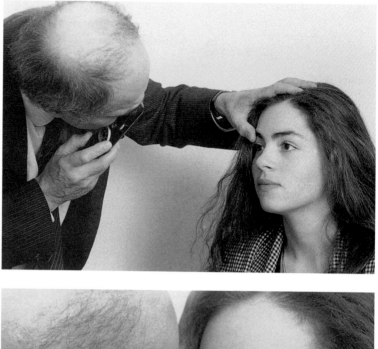

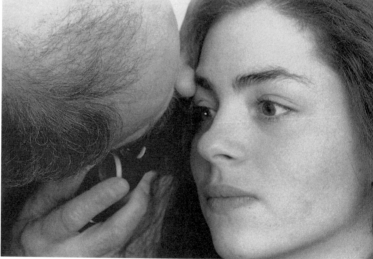

gland. There is less chance that the pupil will constrict and
of course no chance at all if dilating drops have been used.

The posterior pole
Three features dominate:

- the optic nerve head
- the macula
- the retinal vessels.

The optic nerve head is also characterized by three
features:

- M – margin
- C – colour
- C – cup.

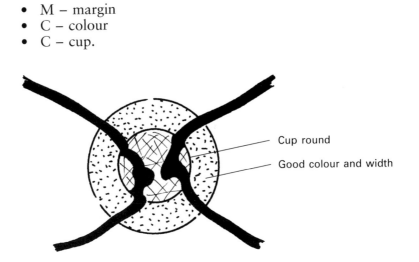

Figure 4.21
The optic nerve head. The vital features are: margin – colour – cup (round is usually physiological and normal)

Cup round

Good colour and width

These aspects will be recalled easily, if we remember that the letters MCC also stand for the nerve head of English cricket which, like that of the eye, accommodates a broad range of appearances that might be taken for normal – sometimes a bit florid, sometimes a bit pale, occasionally a trifle cupped, from time to time blurred round the edges, or maybe just remnants lingering.

The **central macular retina**, with the fovea at the middle, covers an area similar to that of the optic nerve head. It lies a disc and a half's width away from the temporal side of the optic nerve and just below the horizontal meridian.

Figure 4.22
The normal fundus. The features to look for are: disc (MCC); macula – round, dark and regular and on the temporal side of the optic nerve head – blood vessels with no variation in arterial calibre or nipping at the arteriovenous (AV) crossings. The fundal landscape, if seen with the direct ophthalmoscope, will be in small circular segments

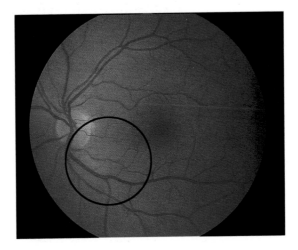

The **arteries** sprout from the optic nerve head to which the darker larger veins return. The vessels on the temporal side, above and below the macula, form the temporal arcade.

Summary
- Is the intraocular pressure raised? (Think aqueous)
- Search for *which part of the eye is affected.* (One-response organ)

Master the seven observations which will indicate which part of the eye is affected:

- central vision for distance
- central vision for near
- field vision
- cornea
- pupil
- anterior chamber
- pressure.

If they do not, they will indicate *which parts are not affected* and provided that

- the field is full, and
- the intraocular pressure is normal, then

the eye is safe and will not deteriorate further without the patient's drawing our attention to that possibility.

The eighth observation, the ophthalmoscope, may help confirm what the first seven have led us to anticipate. Then and only then, do we consider which process from the catalogue of pathology could have given rise to whatever we have found.

Such an unchanging system mastered at brain stem level applies to all other branches of medicine. It applies to the eye as well.

5

Change of appearance

Symptoms come:

- alone
- as a dominant member of a group
- as one amongst equals.

Change of appearance, particularly over a long period, may be so subtle as to be undetected particularly by the one whose appearance is changing. Although old photographs sometimes preserve images not recognizable to every subject, they are often the best way of giving the lie or confirmation to allegations of change.

DRYNESS OF THE SKIN AND EYEBROW THINNING

In the older age groups, such is the classic description of an underactive thyroid. The onset is so insidious, that whilst it may escape near associates, the scaly skull and dull inertia usually shock long lost but recently discovered relatives.

STARING EYES

Retraction of the upper eyelid due to thyroid induced activity of the autonomic levator muscle exposes white sclera above the upper limbus.

PROMINENT EYES

When available space in the orbits ceases to be adequate to contain the eyeballs as well as the orbital contents, then the eyes will advance, pushing the lids aside. This proptosis or exophthalmos is another example of insidious change that may only be noticed by people who have not been around to be unaware of its quiet development.

Figure 5.1
Proptosis. The eyelid occupying too anterior a position prevents the lids from closing. The contents of the orbital apex may compress the optic nerve

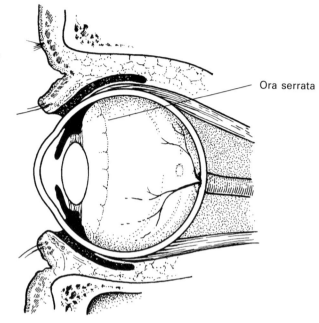

Ora serrata

Whilst such bilateral enlargement has to be regarded as evidence of thyrotoxicosis, we must remember that 20% of cases are unilateral.

Figure 5.2
Exophthalmos. Accumulation of abnormal tissue within the orbit takes up space normally occupied by the eye which responds by occupying a more anterior position. The dangers are: compression of the optic nerve at the orbital apex and exposure of the cornea

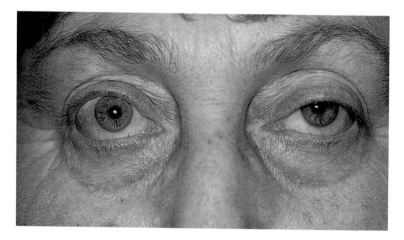

It carries with it two dangers of significance to the eye:

- exposure of the cornea
- compression of the optic nerve at the apex of the orbit.

Action

In the short term corneal exposure can be relieved by:

- Ocular lubricants or artificial tears.
- A lateral tarsorrhaphy narrows the palpebral aperture, reducing exposure and irritation.
- The upper eyelid can be lowered surgically by section of the autonomic levator.

High doses of systemic corticosteroids can frequently reduce the volume of the orbital contents.

Should these drugs fail, then decompression of the orbit by removal of one of the orbital walls is the only way to reduce pressure and preserve vital structures.

ONE SIDED PROTRUSION OF THE EYE

This must always be taken seriously. A mass within the muscle cone produces forward movement (axial proptosis). A mass outside the muscle cone will displace the eye in any direction and is more likely to present with double vision before actual swelling is noted.

If the superior orbital fissure is involved, then there is more than ocular nerve compression to consider. Motor disturbance follows involvement of the third, fourth and sixth cranial nerves whilst sensation on the face and cornea are disturbed by involvement of the trigeminal.

Examination

Computerized tomography
The CT scan has revolutionized the investigation of intracranial and orbital disorders; contrast enhancement can help also in the identification of vascular lesions.

Figure 5.3
Axial CT scan Exophthalmos due to enlargement of extraocular muscles, particularly medial rectus. Optic nerve elongated

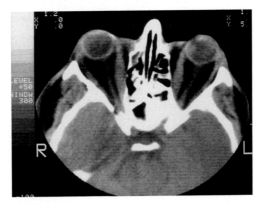

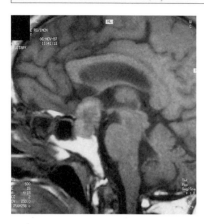

Figure 5.4
Mid line sagittal MRI scan without
contrast: pituitary mass expanding
upwards into the chiasmatic cistern;
encroachment into third ventricular,
optic and infundibular recesses

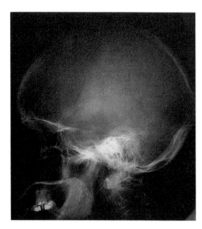

Figure 5.5
Enlarged pituitary fossa X-ray

Magnetic resonance imaging (MRI)

Such imaging is at its best in the uncovering of soft tissue change.

Radiography

Plain films of the skull, although going out of fashion, can give information about enlargement of the stella without the need for excessive radiation.

Although thyroid imbalance has to be the first thought, we have also to consider:

- tumours arising from any of the tissues within the orbit
- inflammatory deposits
- sinus mucoceles
- vascular malformations
- pseudo tumour
- the impression of proptosis due to
  (a) high myopia
  (b) infantile glaucoma
  (c) lid retraction.

Action

An ophthalmic opinion in due course may result in:

- observation for progression
- systemic corticosteroids for thyroid exophthalmos or pseudo tumour
- further referral to a neuro- or maxillo-facial surgeon.

ACUTE PROTRUSION OF ONE EYE IN CHILDHOOD

Rhabdomyosarcoma

A rapidly progressive swelling within the orbit almost always results from this lethal tumour, although happily on occasions it may prove to be due to infection.

Orbital cellulitis

This acute infection of the orbit is either the result of a blood borne disorder in a vulnerable person or the spread of infection from an adjacent sinusitis. The diagnosis is made from:

- all the local signs of inflammation
- systemic fever.

Figure 5.6
Orbital cellulitis

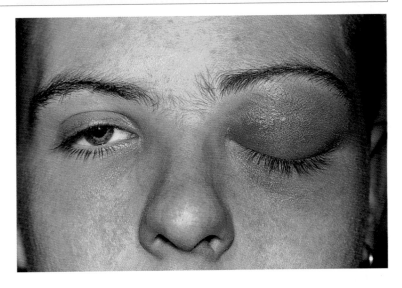

Examination

If the eyelids can be opened, the seven signposts lead to nothing abnormal.

Action

Intensive systemic antibiotics.

ACUTE PROTRUSION OF BOTH EYES

Cavernous sinus thrombosis
This rare and devastating catastrophe which produces gross venous congestion and disturbance of the adjacent:

- third
- fourth
- fifth and
- sixth cranial nerves.

The patient will be clearly prostrated by a severe illness and this is no time to debate trifles at length by the bedside.

Examination

- The extraocular muscles will be paralysed (cranial nerve examination).
- The pupil will be non-reacting.

Action

Urgent, intensive systemic antibiotics.

DROOPING OF THE EYELID

When the upper lid fails to rise above the pupil line the explanation must vary with the age, mode of onset and any companion symptoms.

Figure 5.7
Ptosis. An eyelid, which may droop for many reasons, can diminish vision if it obscures the pupil line

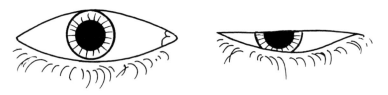

Congenital

In children the complaint is not so much of a change of appearance but rather the parental realization that an appearance present since birth is in fact not standard. A dropped lid in these circumstances is usually brought about by an isolated dystrophy of the levator muscle because both contraction and relaxation are affected.

Aquired ptosis

Third nerve palsy
Discussed under the cranial nerves.

Bilateral drooping of the upper lid
Usually the result of passing time, when so many things begin to droop.

Examination

The seven observations find nothing of consequence.

Action

If the lids are interfering with vision then they can be raised surgically.

DROOPING LIDS THAT DROOP MORE DURING THE DAY

Myasthenia gravis

The hallmark of this condition is a tendency for striated muscle to develop fatigue after repeated action – a state of affairs that improves with rest. It results from the destruction of acetylcholine at the myoneural junction.

Test

Intravenous edrophonium chloride (Tensilon) rapidly relieves the ptosis and confirms the diagnosis of myaesthenia gravis.

Action

Oral pyridostigmine relieves the symptoms. Removal of the thymus can occasionally augment the general improvement.

UNILATERAL DROOPING OF THE LID AND A SMALL PUPIL

Horner's syndrome

The complaint of a dropped lid with the discovery of a constricted pupil brings us into the realms of paralysis of the cervical sympathetic and a subject which will be discussed under pupil abnormalities.

Figure 5.8
Horner's syndrome right eye: dropped lid, small pupil, diminished tear secretion

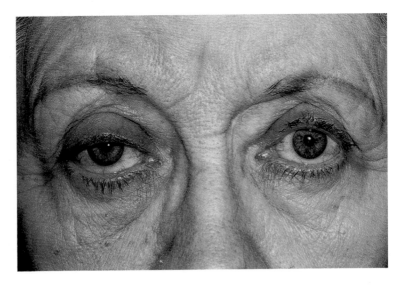

EYELID TUMOURS

Such lumps are common and more so as the years go by.

Papilloma

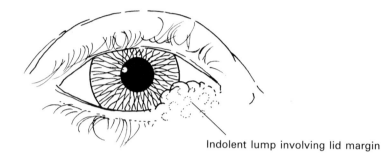

Indolent lump involving lid margin

The most frequent benign lid tumour appears in two forms:

- squamous papilloma
- senile verruca.

Xanthelasma

A common condition resulting in yellow deposits underneath the superficial skin. They may be associated with elevated serum lipids but usually are not.

Haemangioma

Capillary haemangioma

This is the most common vascular malformation. It may develop at birth or not long afterwards, growing rapidly and disappearing spontaneously by about the age of six or seven. Its vascular origin will be demonstrated by bright redness in the more superficial lesions and a darker blue for the deeper ones.

Cavernous haemangioma

These large vascular channels lined with endothelium tend to arise in the teenage years. They do not usually regress and if troublesome require to be removed.

Malignant tumours

The most common are:

- basal cell carcinoma (rodent ulcer)
- squamous cell carcinoma.

The latter can metastasize and both require complete removal.

Rodent ulcer

The hallmark is a dimpled lump with rolled edges and always apparently in the grip of some indolent or recurrent infection from which it never seems to escape.

Figure 5.10
Rodent ulcer: a crusted lump with rolled edges that appears chronically infected and continually and relentlessly growing

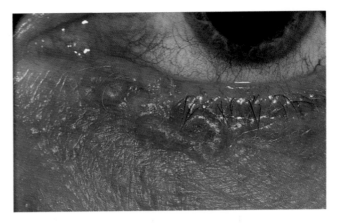

It is not called rodent for nothing, and has the potential to nibble away to extinction all adjacent structures.

Action

Radiotherapy offers as much hope of success as does complete surgical excision with less discomfort. However, with both methods we have to remember the possibility of damage to the lacrimal puncta and the canaliculi and, in the upper lid particularly, radiotherapy threatens permanent obstruction of the tiny ducts carrying tears from the tear gland into the upper conjunctival fornix.

Squamous cell carcinoma

It can spread to regional lymph nodes. Nothing very much distinguishes it from a benign tumour other than its continued growth and tendency to ulceration.

Figure 5.11
Squamous cell carcinoma. Distinguished from the more common papilloma by increasing size and occasional surface ulceration

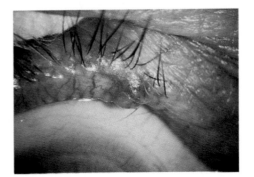

Action

Full excision confirmed by histology.

Jaundice

The serum bilirubin can rise for many reasons but at a pathological level will be most evident in a yellow staining of the normally white scleral conjunctiva.

6

Pain

PAIN IN THE EYE

This section might reasonably start with a couplet that owes more of its elegance and rhythm to William McGonigall than to Alexander Pope

> If pain in the eye is caused by the eye,
> We don't have to search for the reason why

– because it will be obvious.
If there are

- no visual symptoms and
- no positive signs from the ophthalmic ritual

then the source of discomfort almost always lies somewhere else.

PAIN ADJACENT TO THE EYE

Pressure on the posterior occipital nerves trapped by poor head posture between the skull and the atlas can produce spontaneous discomfort right in the forehead.

Temporal arteritis
Aching in the temples, the gums and the jaws together with

- tenderness over the temporal arteries, and
- a raised ESR

are common warning associations of imminent ischaemic optic neuropathy.

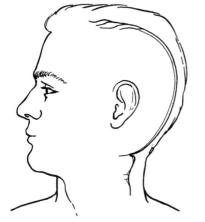

Figure 6.1
The distribution of the posterior occipital nerves. Entrapment between the skull and the atlas, can result in pain in the forehead

PAIN ON MOVING THE HEAD DOWN

Increase in discomfort when the level of the head drops below that of the heart is diagnostic of sinusitis. The pain can be fearful.

Action

- Decongestant nasal sprays.
- Systemic antibiotics if the problem is acute.

PAIN ON WAKING

Headache, worse in the morning can be suggestive of an intracranial tumour. The discomfort may lighten when rising reduces intracranial pressure but tumour headaches would be present every morning, with each episode worse than the last.

PAIN WITH HALOES

Aching in the forehead with blurred vision and haloes made up of all the colours of the rainbow means acute angle closure.

Figure 6.2
The origin of rainbow haloes. The cornea in angle closure, like a fishmonger's window hosed with water, splits light into all the colours of the spectrum

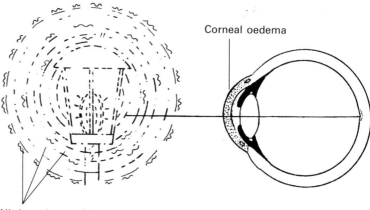

Corneal oedema

All the colours of the visible spectrum

The threat of angle closure is not a disease until it happens. It is a shape. Eyes at risk are usually long-sighted because such eyes are small. Their anterior chambers are shallow, with no room for the pupil to dilate. Nothing happens until circumstances make closure of the angle possible. The sympathetic dilator pulls the pupil backwards against the lens. Aqueous builds up behind the blocked pupil and pushes the iris forwards close to the drainage angle thus preventing aqueous from reaching the normal trabecular meshwork.

Figure 6.3
Block to the aqueous flow at the pupil margin is the first step to angle closure

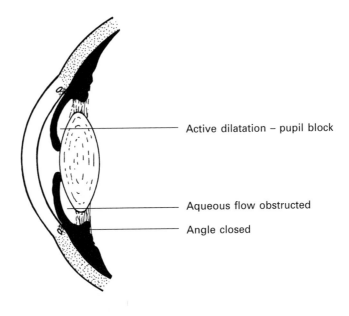

Active dilatation – pupil block

Aqueous flow obstructed

Angle closed

It has to start with dilatation of the pupil which occurs:

- because of the sympathetic activity
- when illumination is diminished at dusk or in the evening.

The cornea becomes waterlogged – hence the haloes and the blurring of vision.

Because the angle closes quickly, the intraocular pressure rises quickly and the patient experiences severe pain in the forehead. The symptoms may be:

- transient, as warning attacks of threatening angle closure and not infrequently misdiagnosed as 'evening migraines', or
- continue as an established attack of acute angle closure.

The eye at risk but not affected
The patient is long-sighted and may have:

- Difficulty with near vision before 40
- A shallow anterior chamber (positive eclipse test)
- No other positive features.

Figure 6.4
The eclipse test. The iris hillock of the shallow anterior chamber is always in shadow on the side remote from the light

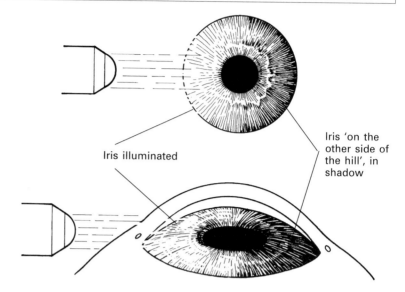

Iris illuminated

Iris 'on the other side of the hill', in shadow

Acute angle closure (acute glaucoma)

- Cloudy vision
- Hazy cornea
- Fixed dilated pupil
- A shallow anterior chamber. If not seen through the hazy cornea then the fellow eye has the same shape.
- The intraocular pressure will be rock hard.

Figure 6.5
Acute angle closure: ciliary injection; fixed dilated pupil; rock hard eye

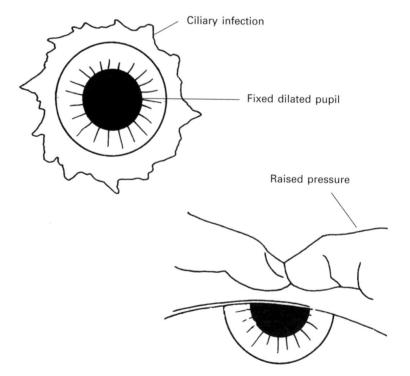

Ciliary infection

Fixed dilated pupil

Raised pressure

PAIN PLUS FLOATERS

The likely cause is inflammation, either of:

- the iris – or
- the whole uveal tract.

It would be unusual for this to happen in a quiet eye.

PAIN ON TOUCH

Tenderness to palpation indicates some form of ocular inflammation – iritis or scleritis – both unusual in a quiet eye.

Figure 6.6
Episcleritis. No general inflammation. A localized area of redness

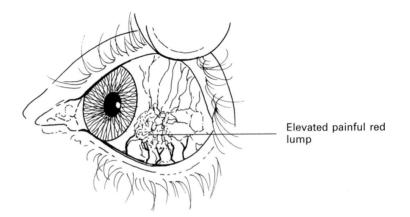

Elevated painful red lump

PAIN ON MOVEMENT

Provided there are symptoms of visual disturbance, the likely cause has to be optic neuritis.

Examination

- Vision diminished.
- Pupil – poorly sustained light reaction.
- The optic nerve head may be
  (a) normal
  (b) swollen
  (c) pale and atrophic from a previous attack.

Inflammation at the optic nerve head will result in a swollen disc. If, however, the inflammation is within the optic nerve itself (retrobulbar neuritis), there will be no sign.

The patient sees little and the doctor sees nothing.

About 50% of patients between 20 and 45 years of age go on to develop multiple sclerosis.

Bilateral optic neuritis can follow viral infection such as measles, influenza or chicken pox.

PAIN AFTER USE

Discomfort in the eyes at such times could point to a refractive error. It could also point to an imbalance of the extraocular muscles (discussed under latent squint).

7

Watering (and discharge)

Tears formed in the tear gland wash over the globe before evaporating or draining into the nose via the nasolacrimal duct. The eye could not survive without tears, but when something is amiss with the lacrimal system a wet eye is what people complain most bitterly about.

There are two kinds of tear production. The first, the basal flow, keeps the external eye moist. The second, the reflex flow, is the response to some disturbance like a foreign body, a finger in the eye or, paradoxically, a dry eye.

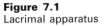

Figure 7.1
Lacrimal apparatus

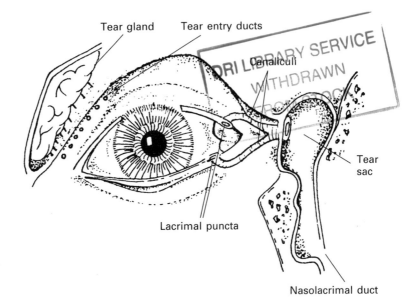

The lids
The lids should contact the globe snugly to allow the punctum access to the tears. Thus, in-turned lids (entropion) or out-turned lids (ectropion), will force any excess tears to dribble over onto the cheek.

BLOCKED NASOLACRIMAL DUCT (IN BABIES)

In babies, the nasolacrimal duct often fails to open fully at birth.

Action

It is best to assume that the block is not permanent. Should watering persist or infection supervene, then probing under general anaesthesia might remove the occluding membrane. If done maladroitly, it may substitute for the transient occlusion a permanent occlusion of its own.

Tear secretion begins some days after birth. Therefore watering at birth, means infection and urgent treatment is necessary.

BLOCKED NASOLACRIMAL DUCT (IN ADULTS)

Blockage may occur following nasal and sinus problems but it would appear in the West to be the price paid for a temperate climate.

If both canaliculi have access to the tear sac then surgery would involve uniting the lacrimal sac to the nasal mucosa through a hole cracked in the bone between the lacrimal fossa and the nasal cavity. Fistulae, which remain so intractable when unwanted, are not so easy to induce surgically and the body will always attempt to block up any unwanted orifices.

Action

Simple measures must precede surgery. Topical astringents like zinc sulphate to the eye with decongestants to the nose can sometimes constrict the duct mucosa at both ends. Prolonged application to the nose ends up doing the reverse.

Unless the patient desires surgery, then there is no indication to refer. Indeed the description of the operation may make most people feel that their symptoms were not really quite as bad as they originally thought.

Acute dacryocystitis

The great reservoir is the lacrimal sac where stagnant tears may explode into a lacrimal abscess – unmistakable as an angry red swelling between the nose and the medial canthus.

Action

In the *short term* systemic antibiotics will usually bring about medical control. The only secure *long term* solution

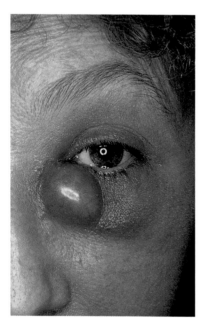

Figure 7.2
Acute dacryocystitis. A painful fiery swelling over the tear gland. Pus may be discharged from the lower canaliculus on pressure

is a dacryocystorhinostomy, which in these circumstances may not appear so repellent an alternative to a lacrimal sac abscess.

RUPTURE OF THE LOWER CANALICULUS (TRAUMA)

Rupture of the canaliculus in the lower lid was a common Friday night injury before seatbelts were enforced by law. Surgical attempts to re-unite the torn ends used to involve arranging them around a silicone tube, which was then passed through the upper canaliculus.

The result was often not only obstruction of the lower canaliculus but obstruction to the upper one as well. Since the upper one has now to do all the work it is best not to threaten its patency in the name of treatment.

Figure 7.3
Laceration of the lower canaliculus. A traumatic cause of intractable watering

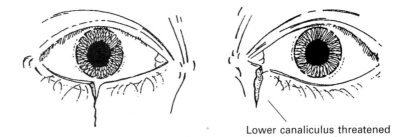

Lower canaliculus threatened

Discharge

Purulent
Watering, augmented by pus, brought about usually by bacterial infection, can occur in the absence of nasolacrimal blockage.

Mucoid
Mucus, rolled into clear strands by the eye lids, tends to collect in the presence of some foreign material, most often stitch ends protruding through the conjunctiva.

8

Disturbance of vision

Visual malfunction, like that of the brain, becomes apparent because of:

- altered behaviour
- features present which should be absent
- features absent which should be present.

ALTERED FUNCTION

When patients talk of distortion, whilst the chiasma (compression) and the cornea (keratoconus) could be to blame, we are almost always thinking of the macula.

Macular degeneration
- Most cases result from age-related macular change –, but
- Not all degeneration is due to age.
  - (a) Myopia – the short-sighted eye is a big eye. Its layers, thinner than standard, occasionally crack. A crack deep to the macula is more common in a young myope than in a normal-sighted person of the same age. Haemorrhage from the choroid then may seep through the crack into the macular retina.
  - (b) An old retinal detachment creeping into the macula may draw attention to itself because of central visual loss. The visual field defect – probably unnoticed by the patient, will be detectable by the doctor if looked for.

Photophobia
Light of an intensity that leaves normal people unaffected may prove too much for:

- eyes deficient in pigment – albinism being the most florid example

Figure 8.1
Opacities, usually in the lens, can cast an orange glow around the light – a halo by any other name – raising the mistaken fear of impending angle closure

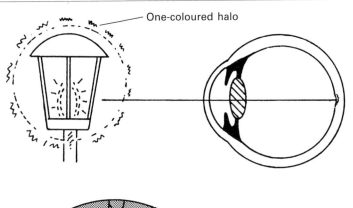

One-coloured halo

Figure 8.2
Myopic fundus. The sclera around the optic nerve head is seen as white through atrophic choroid and pigment retina

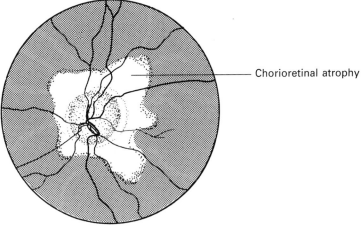

Chorioretinal atrophy

Figure 8.3
A slow detachment can be stopped for a while by spontaneous black lines of chorioretinal adhesions (tide marks). Months or years later it catches the macula and is then an emergency

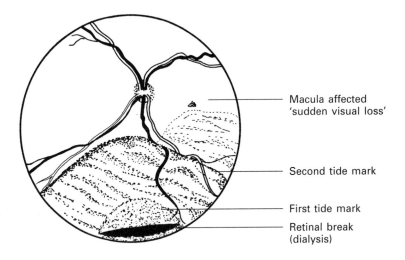

Macula affected 'sudden visual loss'

Second tide mark

First tide mark

Retinal break (dialysis)

- children with infantile glaucoma
- eyes already disturbed by some inflammatory condition such as iritis
- people whose central vision is sensitive for other reasons
  (a) generalized viral infections

(b) infection localized to a particular tissue – e.g. the meninges.

Popular folklore portrays drug dealers, mafiosi and neurotics making public their desire for privacy behind opaque sunglasses. They are not photophobic.

ABNORMAL FEATURES PRESENT

Haloes

Media that are translucent instead of transparent scatter a luminous ring of light around an original light source, as do clouds on a frosty night around the moon.

When the clouds are in the eye and not the sky, they produce two kinds of haloes.

One colour

An opacity, usually in the lens (cataract) bends passing light into a one-coloured ring. Patients will not distinguish one-colour haloes from rainbow haloes unless we ask them and if we do not ask them we will not make the distinction either.

Spectral colours

Figure 8.4
A cornea suddenly oedematous from episodes of angle closure, splits light into the visible spectrum, rainbow haloes raising the genuine fear of impending angle closure

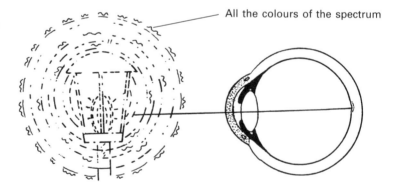

All the colours of the spectrum

A narrow angle can obstruct the aqueous circulation. The cornea, flooded with water, breaks up white light as does the sky after a rain storm. A narrow angle is a shape and is not a disease until the pupil, dilating in conducive circumstances, makes it one. The advance and retreat of warning symptoms take the form of transient haloes, frontal headaches and blurred vision in reduced illumination.

Flashing lights (photopsiae)

Flashing lights alone
Part affected: the retina—Because the retina is light specific, it responds to every disturbance by giving a sensation of light – the most sophisticated of which is normal vision. Occasional flashing with no other symptoms can be brought about by movement of the eyes – a sense of light awareness, seen often only in the dark.

The chorioretinal scarring of successful retinal surgery in itself can produce occasional traction on the retina which in turn brings about flashes of light. These may go on for years.

Flashing lights with headache
Part affected: the intracranial visual pathway—The coruscations of migraine flicker in the half visual field of one side – the nasal field of one eye and the temporal field of its fellow. They are produced by vascular constriction along the optic radiations and in extreme circumstances may produce a complete homonymous hemianopia (loss of the nasal field of one eye and the temporal field of the other). To the patient inexpert in sub-divisions of symptoms, these still merit the name light flashing and on the surface it is little different from any other. A prostrating headache on the same side, presumably due at this stage to vascular dilatation, completes the classic sequence.

Figure 8.5
The visual pathway stretches from the retina to the occipital cortex. Behind the chiasma disturbances catch the homonymous field of both eyes

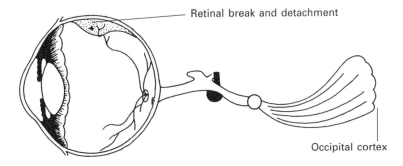

Retinal break and detachment

Occipital cortex

Like all classic sequences it is not as common as the exceptions. The lights can occur without the headache and the headache without the lights. The significant point is the distribution *in the half visual field of one side rather than the whole visual field of one eye.*

Flashing lights with floaters
Flashing lights with floaters are not so very different from floaters with flashing lights, under which heading they will be discussed.

Floaters

To casual observation, all floaters appear the same. It is their companions that reveal potential differences.

Simple

The vitreal gel, liquefying with age, allows previously invisible fibrils to coalesce into those little wisps and tendrils that are so distressing when they first appear.

Floaters with flashing lights (neither dominating)

Posterior vitreal detachment—A fashionable name given to flashing lights and floaters when no retinal break can be found to explain them. There is no firm sequence, no loss of vision and the sudden activity becomes less of a flurry over a few days.

Figure 8.6
Detachment of the posterior vitreous. A popular diagnosis even when it has not happened

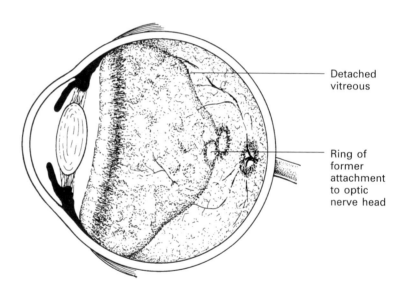

Detached vitreous

Ring of former attachment to optic nerve head

A true posterior separation is recognized by the fibrous ring which marks the attachment of the posterior vitreous to the optic nerve head. But even that does not mean that the whole vitreous has separated. There is more than a touch of the Emperor's clothes between the public diagnosis and the private wonder at just what exactly is wrong.

Floaters preceded by flashing lights

Retinal break—As with thunder and lightning, it is the lightning that comes first. Traction by the vitreous abnormally adherent to the retina produces, quite predictably, flashes of light. As the traction continues, the retina tears and the flashing stops. A shower of floaters now dominates and the sequence of *lights first and floaters second* is critical.

Figure 8.7
The origin of the horseshoe break.
Vitreal traction on the retina begins
with light flashing, which stops
when the retina tears amidst a
shower of floaters

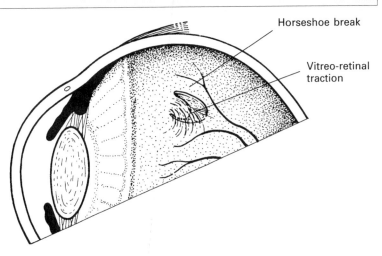

Horseshoe break

Vitreo-retinal
traction

*Floaters preceded by light flashing and followed by a
shadow*
Retinal break plus detachment—In addition to the symptoms described under retinal break, liquefied vitreous passes
through into the sub-retinal space producing a retinal
separation and a flickering shadow in the corresponding
field of vision.

Figure 8.8
The origin of a retinal detachment.
The two prerequisites are a
detached liquid vitreous and a hole
in the retina

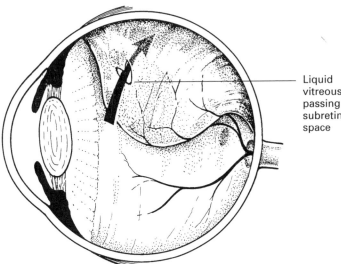

Liquid
vitreous
passing into
subretinal
space

Floaters and visual loss – sudden
Part affected

- Macula – central loss.
- Vitreous – general loss.

Haemorrhage at the macula can be found in:

- age related disciform degeneration
- myopia.

Vitreal haemorrhage, arising possibly from:

- hypertension
- diabetic retinopathy
- haemorrhagic retinopathy, due either to
  (a) some vasculo-occlusive disease
  (b) no recognizable cause
  (c) generalized bleeding disorders
  (d) aspirin or warfarin
  (e) a macro-aneurysm – rarely.

Figure 8.9
Vitreal haemorrhage. Traction tearing the retina may also tear a retinal blood vessel

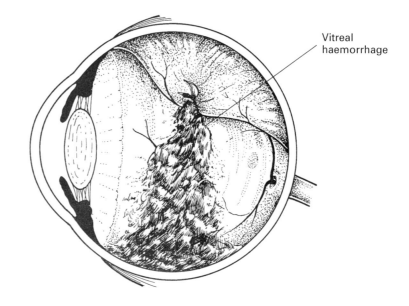

Vitreal haemorrhage

In the absence of a recognized reason for bleeding, a retinal break (with or without a retinal detachment) must be assumed.

The presence of a frank detachment might be recognized by:

- field loss detectable with the hands, or by,
- poor projection of light.

Floaters and general loss – gradual
Part affected: vitreous—Floaters always mean something in the vitreous and this sort of presentation is very suggestive of an inflammatory vitritis arising from the choroid or as

part of a general inflammation of the uveal tract. The vision is slightly affected.

A fine dispersal of opacities through the vitreous dulls the red reflex, and the general view of the retina with the direct ophthalmoscope is even more blurred than usual.

NORMAL FEATURES ABSENT

Transient absence of vision (amaurosis fugax)

Part affected: Blood supply to the optic nerve—The complaint is of a sudden onset of clouding out of vision which, after some minutes, may clear to normal. The exact nature of the loss can indicate whether the cause be:

- hypotension, or
- embolization.

Hypotension

Loss of vision begins from the periphery inwards and clears in the reverse direction. Such episodes arise because the blood flow of the eye diminishes. The cause is either:

- postural – where the head rises faster than its blood supply (this would be obvious from the history), or
- carotid insufficiency on the same side as the symptoms – by far the commonest. This can be confirmed by
  (a) poor pulsation of the affected carotid artery
  (b) a bruit detected with a stethoscope over the same vessel.

Figure 8.10
Amaurosis fugax. Narrowing of the internal carotid can result in hypotensive field loss – darkening from the periphery inwards; clearing in the reverse direction

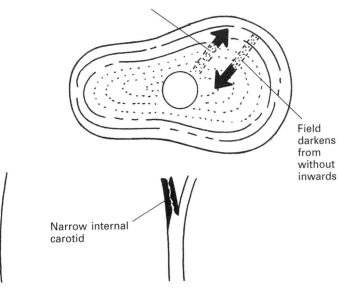

Field clears from within outwards

Field darkens from without inwards

Narrow internal carotid

Embolization

The loss is described as a curtain either coming from above or below. The emboli must have a source in the vascular tree, and if large the loss will not be transient.

Cholesterol plaques feature prominently in textbook descriptions of the retinal arterioles – little glistening dots, lodging at the vascular bifurcations. They do not feature so prominently in the clinical appearances picked up by occasional ophthalmoscopists.

Progressive reduction of vision

Such complaints almost always refer to the centre. Loss of field alone is rarely noticed.

Part affected: optic nerve (up to the chiasma)—The most common causes from the inventory of pathology would be:

*   compression
*   trauma (late effect).

The symptoms of optic nerve disease are frequently described by the patients as a sensation of looking through a filter.

Colour perception

When conduction along the optic nerve is damaged, by say compression or demyelination, the retina supplied by the affected fibres does not perceive the colour red as the brilliant hue perceived by the unaffected retina. In the presence of red/green deficiency, the contrast between the brilliance of whatever colour is perceived by the normal retina and the duller version served by the damaged fibres is equally valid.

Figure 8.11
The Mutlukan–Cullen test.
Diminished perception of red follows the conduction defects in the optic nerve which themselves sometimes follow compression or demyelination

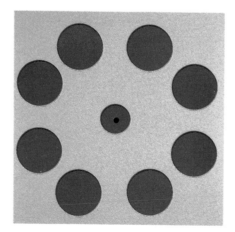

The Mutlukan–Cullen Test (1991, and available through *Optometry Today*) is essentially a card with a series of dots circling the fixation point. Its inexpensive simplicity, which ought to lead to its universal adoption, will doubtless do the opposite.

Equal perception of red at identical points around fixation would suggest that the optic nerve is not involved. Conversely, a decline in intensity of perception to one side or the other would suggest that it is.

Permanent diminution of vision

Lazy eye (amblyopia)

Such an eye is to all intents and purposes normal. It has never been allowed to develop central vision.

Loss of dark adaptation

Night blindness is not a term that most people would use but they might admit on questioning that the vision does not adapt to the dark when the lights go out.

The most common cause is following widespread photocoagulation for diabetes. Happily rarer though more tragic causes are retinitis pigmentosa and inherited retinal degeneration, which will eventually leave the patient with a tunnel of central vision in a field of darkness.

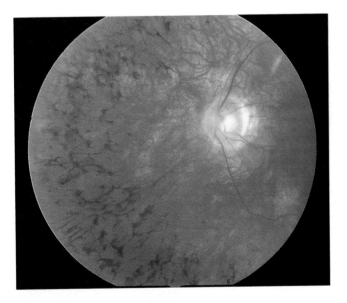

Figure 8.12
Retinitis pigmentosa – the most celebrated of the retinal degenerations. Characterized by: night blindness; field constriction; a scatter of pigment over the posterior retina in the form of bone corpuscles

Most patients rarely recognize the presence of field loss, and even in those who do we should look first at heavy spectacle frames and drooping upper eyelids before thinking of anything more sinister.

9

Loss of vision

Most textbooks deal with visual loss as a catalogue of pathology, brightened with a clinical touch, a scatter of symptoms, a dash of epidemiology and the inevitable tableau of retina spreading across every page. Add an obscuring wash of ophthalmic jargon and the mystification is complete. What the patient complains of is concealed in the description of a condition which we cannot identify until we know what the complaint actually is.

Dilating drops are withheld for fear that chronic glaucoma might somehow suddenly turn into acute glaucoma and the ophthalmoscope goes on to produce its customary blur.

Explanations will not flutter about the ophthalmoscope like moths just because we have switched on the light. However, a chrysalis of suspicion can develop into a fully fledged diagnosis if we go through the ophthalmic ritual, step by step, using the ophthalmoscope only to confirm what we already know.

Visual loss may be either *total* or *partial*, in *one eye* or *both eyes, sudden* or *gradual*.

TOTAL LOSS – ONE EYE – SUDDEN

The cause must be occlusion of:

- the central retinal artery, or
- the arterioles of the optic nerve and optic nerve head.

Findings

- No light perception.
- The affected pupil does not respond directly to light (inflow defect).

Figure 9.1
Central retinal arterial occlusion – the cherry red spot. The macula dimples and hollows to its absolute centre where, even in its oedematous state, it allows the redness of the choroid to shine through when it is masked by oedema everywhere else

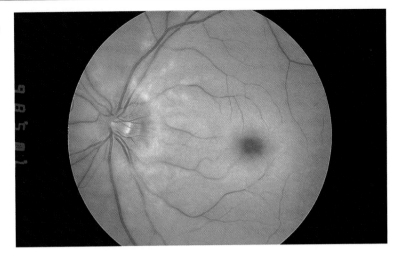

- The disc may be pale and swollen (ischaemic optic neuropathy) – the retina may be creamy white except for the cherry spot at the macula.

Hypertension, diabetes, arteriosclerosis or a source of embolism must always be considered in the older age, groups particularly, temporal arteritis must be the first thought.

Pain in the temple is commonly described as an associate of temporal arteritis but generalized headaches and pains in the gums or jaws are just as common. The matter is one of extreme urgency because the condition can strike the second eye whilst we are slowly debating the need for swift action over the first. Its remote cousin – polymyalgia rheumatica – may lurk in the shadows with no locating symptoms of any kind until it is too late.

Figure 9.2
Distribution of the temporal artery – where tenderness may be felt in temporal arteritis

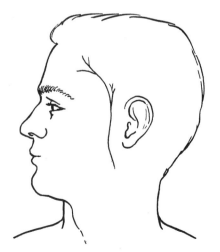

Action

- Reduction of the intraocular pressure with intravenous acetazolamide (500 mg) can sometimes allow the artery to re-open. *Urgent referral may allow the early tapping of aqueous from the anterior chamber for a more rapid reduction of pressure.*
- If arteritis be suspected, then treatment must be commenced immediately with systemic corticosteroids – prednisolone 40 mg daily.

An erythrocyte sedimentation rate (ESR) of below 45 mm in the first hour makes the diagnosis unlikely. If it is above that level then a temporal artery biopsy will confirm or refute the diagnosis.

Aspirin – 75 mg daily – is prescribed almost routinely, in the hope that it will prevent any embolic episodes.

PARTIAL LOSS – ONE EYE – SUDDEN

Patient's complaint	Condition
I Sudden uniform dulling of vision with no other symptoms	**Occlusion of the central retinal vein (or branch)**
II Central loss with pain on ocular movement	**Optic neuritis**
III Flashing lights, floaters, flickering shadow in the vision followed by localized loss	**Retinal detachment**
IV A uniform swarm of floaters suddenly blacking out vision	**Vitreal haemorrhage**
V Inadvertent closure of the good eye revealing	**Sudden awareness of long standing poor vision**

I CENTRAL RETINAL VEIN OCCLUSION (CRVO)

Findings

- Visual acuity is usually reduced to finger counting (CF).
- The pupil demonstrates an inflow defect.
- The stormy sunset retina, with its turmoil of flame haemorrhages and swollen veins, is unmistakable.

If by some lucky chance ischaemia is not a major element, then central vision will be spared and so will the pupil reaction. However, it is usual for this occlusion to be accom-

Figure 9.3
Central retinal vein occlusion – the stormy sunset of central vision – an associate of: chronic simple glaucoma; hypertension; diabetes; hyperviscosity

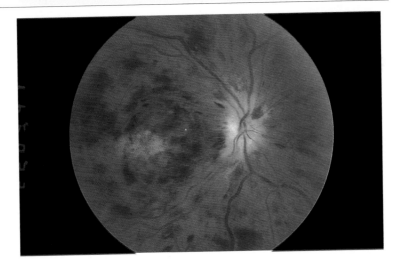

panied by ischaemia and the standard ocular response to ischaemia, whatever the cause (one-response organ), is to develop new blood vessels where they are not wanted:

- on the optic nerve head, and
- in the angle between the iris and the cornea.

Vessels from the optic nerve head may bleed into the vitreal cavity. Vessels in the angle block the trabecular meshwork and acutely raise the pressure of the eye with pain and inflammation. The process takes some 3 months to develop, a time lapse remembered as the 100 day glaucoma.

Action

- Diabetes and hypertension are both well known for their ill effects on the circulation.
- Increased blood viscosity makes thrombosis more likely.
- The chronic raised pressure of long standing glaucoma can impede the venous blood flow.

Should the 100 day glaucoma threaten, then the widespread induction of chorioretinal scars with a laser may help prevent the development of new blood vessels. The aim of this treatment, as in diabetes, is to destroy poorly perfused retinal tissue, to destroy the metabolic impulse to new blood vessel formation and to induce regression of any vessels that have already formed.

II Branch retinal vein occlusion (BRVO)

- Central vision frequently disturbed.

- The fundal picture is essentially a localized version of the stormy sunset.

Action

It is sometimes possible for a line of laser burns to roll back the oedema from the central retina with a dramatic improvement in visual function.

II OPTIC NEURITIS

Sudden visual loss together with pain and movement of the eye is a classic description of retrobulbar or optic neuritis. They differ only in their position. The signs of optic neuritis are visible at the optic nerve head. Those of retrobulbar neuritis are hidden within the optic nerve itself.

Findings

- Visual acuity may be reduced below finger counting (CF) to hand movements (HM) – or less.
- The pupil responds very sluggishly or not at all to direct light on the affected side (inflow defect).
- The disc may be swollen (optic neuritis) or normal (retrobulbar neuritis).

Action

Reassurance that the vision will return almost to its original level can generally be given.

It is not necessary to say that there is a 50% chance of eventual multiple sclerosis – particularly if the symptoms worsen with exercise.

Figure 9.4
The retina, normally transparent when flat, is grey in profile when detached

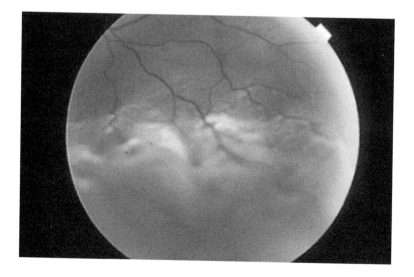

There is no known treatment for unilateral optic neuritis. Drugs given, whilst coincidental with remission, may be given credit they do not deserve. Remote picturesque clinics, offering hope and worthless remedies, flourish as the condition goes through one of its periodic bouts of spontaneous improvement.

Referral the next day will at least give some comfort whilst the vision improves without treatment.

III RETINAL DETACHMENT

- Flashing lights.
- Floaters.
- A sudden flickering in the field of vision.

Findings

There is a higher incidence of retinal detachment in myopes but it can occur after cataract extraction, after long forgotten injury, or spontaneously as well.

- Visual acuity may be normal if the central area is not yet involved.
- Loss of field will correspond to the area of the detachment.
- A grey rippling reflex will take the appearance of the normal red reflex.

Action

This is an ophthalmic emergency, particularly if the macula is intact.

IV VITREAL HAEMORRHAGE

Sudden loss together with:

- a swarm of heavy floaters
- simultaneous visual loss
- possibly flashing lights.

In the absence of diabetes, hypertension and the generalized bleeding disorders, the vitreal haemorrhage must be presumed due to a retinal break. There may well be an associated retinal detachment, both obscured by the haemorrhage.

- Visual acuity may be reduced to light perception (PL).
- The pupil responds briskly to direct light.
- A black reflex will obscure the normal red reflex.

Figure 9.5
Vitreal haemorrhage. In the absence
of other bleeding disorders, likely to
be associated with a retinal break
and/or a retinal detachment

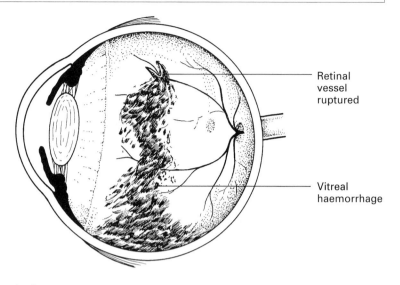

Retinal
vessel
ruptured

Vitreal
haemorrhage

Action

This is a qualified emergency. Referral the next day is
mandatory unless the cause, such as repeated bleeding from
diabetic retinopathy, is already well known.

V SUDDEN AWARENESS OF LONG STANDING POOR VISION

The incidental closure of one good eye can give the impression of sudden failure in a fellow eye that has been defective for years. It must not be assumed that all such eyes have
been lazy since birth.

Action

There are many possible causes but only one examination
ritual.

APPARENT PARTIAL LOSS – ONE EYE – SUDDEN

Homonymous hemianopia
Most people have never imagined that both eyes contribute
to the vision of one side. Because the temporal field is wider
than the nasal field, the eye with the temporal loss is always
blamed.
   *The usual history is of loss in one eye, which questioning
and examination reveal to be actually of one side (both eyes
affected).*

Findings

• Visual acuity may be normal.

Figure 9.6
Homonymous hemianopia. The
visual pathway behind the chiasma
on one side serves the visual field
on the other side

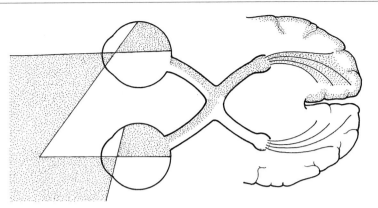

- The fields will show an equal defect to the same side of the fixation point in each eye.
- The cause is usually a vascular accident behind the chiasma, and if behind the mid-brain it will leave the pupil reflexes intact.

Action

- Hypertension, diabetes and blood disorders must again be excluded, and
- a source of embolus must be sought.

Treatment of the underlying circulatory disorder and if necessary regular aspirin may help prevent a similar disaster in the other field.

PARTIAL LOSS – BOTH EYES – SUDDEN

BILATERAL OPTIC NEURITIS
The appearances of bilateral optic neuritis are identical to those when only one eye is affected. Bilateral inflammation, however, is much more likely to follow some generalized viral infection.

Action

Post viral optic neuritis can be shortened with a sharp course of systemic corticosteroids starting with 60 mg of prednisolone daily, reducing over 10 days.

PARTIAL LOSS– ONE EYE – GRADUAL

I   Creeping (usually) inferior retinal detachment.
II Choroidal melanoma.

I Creeping retinal detachment

The cause is often a congenital weakness in the peripheral retina or a long forgotten injury. It may be noticed only when the lifting retina catches the macula thus reducing the central vision. Creeping field loss is usually asymptomatic.

Figure 9.7
Retinal detachment – a surgical emergency

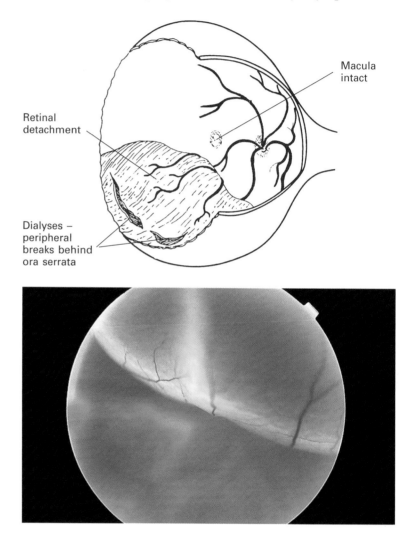

Macula intact

Retinal detachment

Dialyses – peripheral breaks behind ora serrata

Findings

- Central loss varies in direct proportion to the duration of macular involvement.
- The field defect corresponds to the area of the detachment.
- A flat grey reflex replaces the red reflex in the lower fundus. (In congenital cases, similar early changes are often found in the other eye.)

Action

The treatment is surgical.

II CHOROIDAL MELANOMA

The presentation is that of a creeping retinal detachment. Fundal examination may reveal anything from a mottled grey black shadow to a round solid dark lump of varying size.

Figure 9.8
Choroidal melanoma, with an annual incidence of one per 100 000, is not always black. A fluid detachment of the retina adjacent to the solid detachment is diagnostic

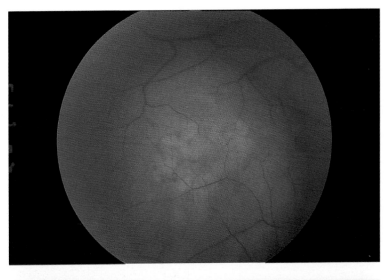

Figure 9.9
A naevus, benign because of its jet blackness and sharp edges. Not uncommon and not uncommonly taken for something sinister

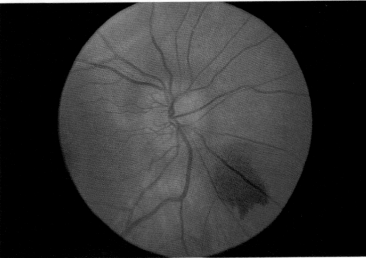

Action

Management has moved forward from the obligatory enucleation of 10 years ago. The tumour can be obliterated by:

- cryocoagulation
- laser coagulation
- generalized radiation
- plaque radiation
- simple excision.

PARTIAL LOSS – BOTH EYES – GRADUAL

Patient's complaint	Condition
I Gradual loss sometimes associated with (i) monocular diplopia (ii) monochromatic haloes (iii) increasing myopia	Cataract
II Central visual loss usually with no other identifying features	Macular degeneration
III No symptoms until late nasal field loss or central retinal vein occlusion	Chronic glaucoma
IV Central loss usually, though occasionally sudden floaters associated with unsuspected maturity onset diabetes	Diabetic retinopathy

I Cataract

Findings

With the pupil dilated, opacities in the lens can be picked up against the red reflex with the ophthalmoscope set at about 24 cm from the eye.

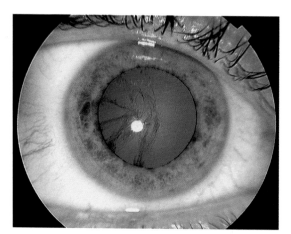

Figure 9.10
Cataract – best seen against the red reflex through the dilated pupil with an ophthalmoscope held some 20 cm away from the eye

Figure 9.11
How to pick up opacities in the clear media

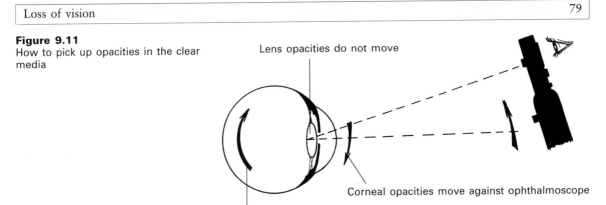

Lens opacities do not move

Corneal opacities move against ophthalmoscope

Vitreal opacities move with ophthalmoscope

Action

Extraction of the cataract and insertion of a lens implant is indicated when the visual defect is interfering with the patient's lifestyle.

II Macular degeneration

Not all macular disturbance is due to age. The macular can be affected by:

- diabetes
- creeping retinal detachment
- hypertension
- anything else from the catalogue of pathology.

Figure 9.12
Degeneration at the macula can take many forms: atrophy; pigmentary disturbance; exudate; haemorrhage

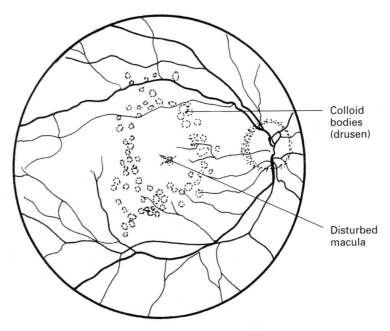

Colloid bodies (drusen)

Disturbed macula

Findings

Through the dilated pupil, the normal dark, round regular appearance of the macula will be broken into:

- patches of atrophy (dry)
- scar formation (dry)
- haemorrhage (wet)
- oedema (wet)
- exudate (may be either).

Action

- For dry degeneration there is no treatment.
- For wet degeneration, intravenous sodium fluorescein can demonstrate points of leakage from one layer of the eye to another. If these points are not directly over the macula, and rarely they are not, they can sometimes be sealed with a laser.
- Treatment of general disorders and removal, if possible, of other causes.

III Chronic glaucoma

A condition that is common and sinister – because it is usually asymptomatic until field vision has been grievously damaged.

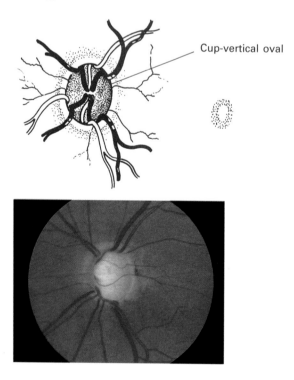

Figure 9.13
Cupped disc – the hallmark of glaucoma, the pathological process

Cup-vertical oval

Findings

- The central visual acuity is not affected until the late stages. The hand movement field, in the late stages, will demonstrate variable loss, particularly on the nasal side.
- The intraocular pressure is usually raised.
- The normal cup of the optic nerve head expands into a vertical oval.
- May present with CRVO.

Action

Discussed under chronic glaucoma.

IV Diabetic retinopathy

Many maturity onset diabetics do not realize they have diabetes. In younger diabetics, duration and poor control rather than severity are the key note in the development of retinal changes. The underlying ischaemic process is also at work in the kidneys and heart and other essential organs.

Findings

The effects of diabetes on the eye are discussed in a separate section.

Action

All diabetics require to have their eyes looked at regularly. Fundal examination must be carried out through the dilated pupil:

- in background retinopathy every year
- in more severe forms every 6 months or more often.

PARTIAL LOSS – BOTH EYES – GRADUAL: SOME UNCOMMON CAUSES

I Hypertensive retinopathy

Hypertension, like glaucoma, is often unsuspected. It should be diagnosed with the sphygmomanometer and not the ophthalmoscope.

Laser photocoagulation and vitrectomy can rescue eyes previously lost because of:

- central or branch retinal vein occlusion
- vitreal haemorrhage.

II Pituitary adenoma

The enlarging pituitary gland causes a variety of conditions but if it compresses the optic chiasma, irregular visual damage will result. If macular fibres at the chiasma are affected, then the central vision will be blunted.

The condition may masquerade as glaucoma without any rise of pressure (low tension glaucoma).

Findings

- The pituitary facies.
- Bi-temporal field loss.
- Dulled awareness of a red target in the affected field.
- Disc pallor due to long compression.

Action

Although no longer fashionable, a lateral radiograph of the skull can very efficiently reveal signs of pituitary enlargement. CT scanning or MRI scanning are more expensively in favour today.

Common things are common and we must remember

- *to ask which part of the eye is affected* (one-response organ)
- *that something may have happened to the aqueous circulation*
- *that field loss may have occurred unsuspected.*

THE REASON WHY

Retinal detachment

The inside of the eye has already been compared to a brandy goblet with an eccentric stem, lined with fine cellophane – attached at the rim and attached at the stem. This cellophane, like the retina, is potentially separable everywhere else. The contents of the goblet are a clear half-set jelly – the vitreous, also attached at the rim and attached at the stem. Occasionally, abnormal adhesions develop between the vitreous and the retina. These adhesions make the retina respond by light flashing which stops when the retina tears, showering the vitreous with a swarm of floaters. If the vitreous now liquefies, it will pass through the retinal break separating from the wall of the eye, recognized by flickering and possibly a shadow in the corresponding field of vision. Cut off from half its blood supply, the retina will starve and in due course become so rigid that replacement will be impossible.

Such is the essence of retinal detachment. The breaks can occur in different places:

Figure 9.14
The layered structure of the eye

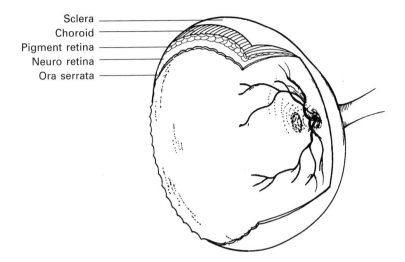

Sclera
Choroid
Pigment retina
Neuro retina
Ora serrata

- on the equator – usually in large myopic eyes
- near the ora (the rim)
  (a) following loss of vitreous during cataract surgery
  (b) dissinsertion of the ora serrata due to injury
  (c) a congenital split in the retina behind an intact ora serrata – dialysis.

The essence of surgery is to find the retinal break(s). An inflammation is induced around where the break will settle with freezing (cryocoagulation). The break is sealed by buckling the ocular layers inwards with silicone rubber or sponge stitched on to the sclera and/or by surface tension induced by an air bubble within the vitreal cavity. A permanent seal is produced as the inflammatory reaction forms a watertight chorioretinal scar.

Figure 9.15
Forward movement of the vitreous, the cause of aphakic retinal detachment, is a rare occurrence today

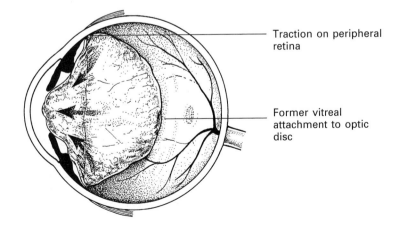

Traction on peripheral retina

Former vitreal attachment to optic disc

Figure 9.16
Freezing applied to a lower retinal
break. If the retina is detached such
inflammation cannot be produced
with a laser.

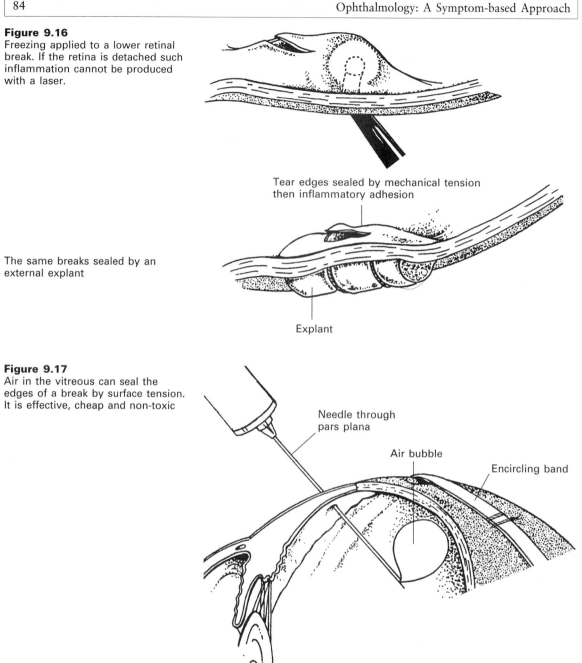

Tear edges sealed by mechanical tension
then inflammatory adhesion

The same breaks sealed by an
external explant

Explant

Figure 9.17
Air in the vitreous can seal the
edges of a break by surface tension.
It is effective, cheap and non-toxic

Needle through
pars plana

Air bubble

Encircling band

Vitrectomy has extended the surgical repertoire in cases
that used to be considered shrunken beyond surgical recall.
The techniques generally involve doing things that were
considered unimaginable in the not very distant past –
cutting out the vitreous, sectioning traction bands, peeling
membranes from the surface of the retina and introducing
silicone oil, heavy liquids, air and long acting gases.

Figure 9.18
Vitrectomy – one of the major
advances in ophthalmic surgery:
makes space in the eye; clears
vitreal opacities; allows intraocular
manipulation

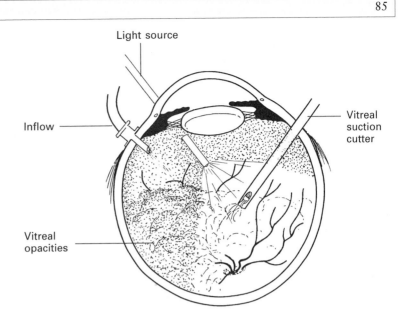

Light source

Inflow

Vitreal
suction
cutter

Vitreal
opacities

The explants sutured to the sclera very occasionally find
their way to the surface of the conjunctiva where, if a source
of irritation, they would have to be removed.

Figure 9.19
An explant eroding the conjunctiva –
yet another cause of acute
conjunctivitis

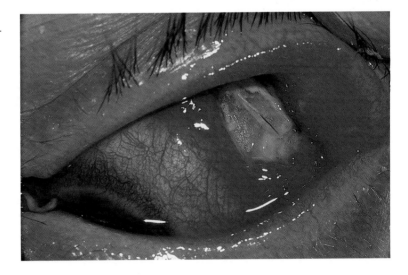

APPARENT VISUAL LOSS

The sudden discovery that the vision in one eye is not as
good as that of the other and the assumption that it must
therefore be of recent origin is far more common than might
be expected. Such eyes may be

• Lazy (amblyopic). They are physically normal but have
  never fully developed central vision. Central vision is not

a birthright but rather a quality that can be stunted if its development is obstructed during the first two or three years of life. Anything that prevents normal images focusing on the retina during these early years will produce amblyopia. Such impediments can be:

(a) dropped eyelid
(b) congenital cataract
(c) childhood squint
(d) an extreme error of refraction often different from that of the fellow eye (anisometropia).

• Damaged in some way, for example with a scar of toxoplasmosis at the macula.

10

Cataract

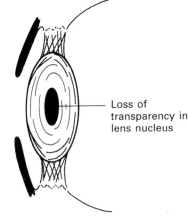

Figure 10.1
Nuclear cataract

Loss of
transparency in
lens nucleus

Cataract is undoubtedly the cause of the majority of referrals. Technically, any opacity in the lens is called a cataract, but it becomes of clinical significance when it interferes with the quality of visual life. The cataract develops in the lens, which, as usual, has one fundamental answer to insult – it becomes opaque.

The lens, although shaped like a lentil, is internally like a transparent plum stone, flesh and skin being equivalent to nucleus, cortex and capsule. This lens forms a critical part of the optical system of the eye. In the past, it was removed completely and replaced with what appeared to be a magnifying glass in a spectacle frame, and the whole arrangement was called aphakia.

The manipulation was optically not unlike taking an essential lens from the middle of a telescope and fitting it on to a bracket at the end. Armed with such an instrument, Admiral Nelson would not have needed to 'clap the glass to his sightless eye,' deliberately to miss the vital signal at the battle of Copenhagen. He could have clapped the glass to either eye and still have missed what he did not want to see. Yet such was the optical arrangement inflicted with surgical pride on all patients with cataract, not so very long ago.

It gave rise to the notion, still current today, that a cataract had to be ripe before extraction could be considered. Technically it makes no difference whether the lens is clear or not. The real reason was that vision after such a cataract extraction was so awful that we had to wait for the vision before surgery to be even worse so that anything we produced would be an improvement.

Lens implants have changed all that. It was found during the last war that pilots tolerated fragments of windscreen Perspex within the eye indefinitely, because they were chemically inert. Out of the misfortune of these brave men, has grown the technique of lens implantation, which restores the

Figure 10.2
Aphakic glasses should now be of historical interest only. The optical impulse behind the search for lens implant

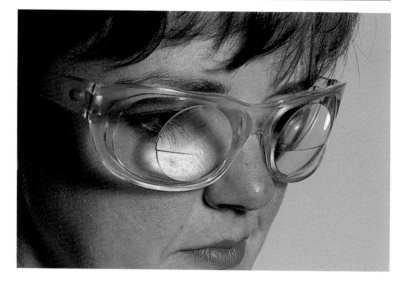

optical balance of the eye in a way unthinkable in those not so far off days, when patients preferred to be happy with poor vision through their own lens than be demented by the 'perfect' vision of aphakia.

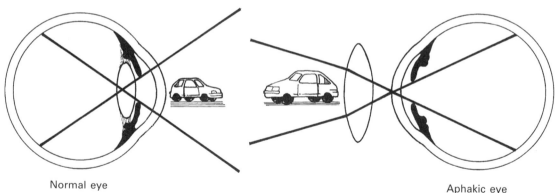

Normal eye   Aphakic eye

Figure 10.3
Normal eye. Normal image. Large field
Aphakic eye. Magnified image. Small field

Before total removal of the lens was technically possible, posterior dislocation of the cataract into the vitreous was the favoured technique of the travelling charlatans – the most famous of whom was the Chevalier Taylor. The lens was toppled swiftly either by a flicked thumbnail or by an actual needle plunged through the pupil and the whole manoeuvre was known as 'couching the cataract'.

Since those cataracts were ripe, like leaking plums in the wasp season, there was a very real danger that the technique would burst them as well. The eye, not recognizing its lens protein as self, would react with a uveitis destructive of the iris and ciliary body. Happily for the Chevalier, the storm clouds did not collect immediately. With the patient's gratitude translated into something more negotiable and indeed negotiated, he would demonstrate his talent for another rapid movement and vanish before the storm broke.

Figure 10.4
Posterior chamber lens implant seen clearly against the red reflex through the dilated pupil

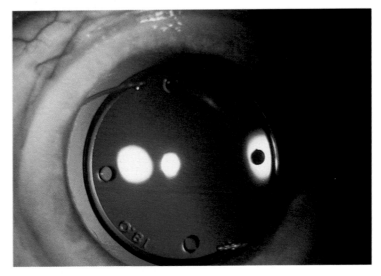

Relief from infirmity has always been a lucrative pursuit for the travelling quack. The Chevalier was no exception and he travelled far in great style. He continually had to.

11

Three serious causes of a red eye

Before we can call an eye abnormal and red, we must first define what we mean by normal and white. The definition is based on conjunctival appearances, which vary with their position.

The sclera is seen as egg-shell white, through the translucent vascular conjunctiva and (in youth) the subconjunctival Tenons capsule. The scleral dominance fades as the conjunctiva folds away under the fornix and then towards the front again where it becomes pinker and pinker until on the deep surface of the lids it has become almost red. So much for the normal.

There is scarcely much more to the abnormal, because there are only three causes of inflammation that could be called serious and they all have one thing in common: *redness dominant around the margin of the cornea.* This inflammation need not look dramatic. Indeed, a good working rule is that the more dramatic an inflammatory episode appears, the less serious it is likely to be.

Figure 11.1
Ciliary injection. The cardinal sign of a serious red eye

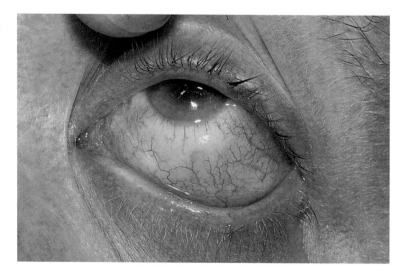

Although this inflammation has many names, the most rational is *ciliary injection*. When the front of the eye is seriously inflamed, the ciliary body is always involved. It extends from the limbus to the insertions of the rectus muscles, and were this area of sclera free of conjunctiva, the blood vessels over its entire surface would be seen to be engorged. Only those adjacent to the cornea are clearly seen because there the sub-conjunctival tissue is at its thinnest. Three serious conditions share this redness dominant around the corneal margin, but each presents in a different way.

Presentation	Condition
• Pain – intense, briefly relieved when the eyelid is lifted away from the eye Watering Vision blurred	**Keratitis (any breach of the corneal epithelium)**
• Discomfort or pain – deep and relieved by nothing Floaters Vision may be blurred	**Iritis**
• Pain in the forehead – prostrating/nauseating Vision – usually severely affected History of rainbow haloes and transient blurring of vision when illumination was reduced – information collected in tranquillity after the very evident cause is dealt with.	**Acute angle closure**

If the inflammation does not dominate around the corneo-scleral limbus, then we are not dealing with one of the major three.

KERATITIS

Abrasion

Usually the result of trauma or when the eyelids opening in the morning have stuck to a vulnerable epithelium overnight (recurrent corneal erosion). The pain and watering is so intense that the eye cannot open sufficiently for any subjective description of vision.

Examination

Sodium fluorescein marks out the area of deficient epithelium.

Figure 11.2
Fluorescein stain, picking up areas of absent corneal epithelium

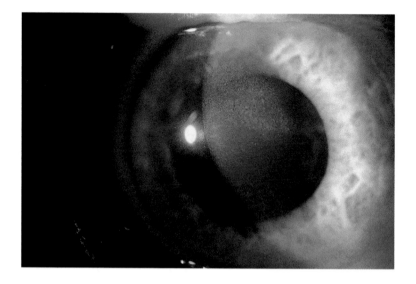

Action

- Topical anaesthesia relieves pain – but continued use delays epithelial regeneration.
- Topical antibiotics – in the presence of any apparent infection.
- Closure of the eyelids with adhesive tape allows the corneal epithelium the best chance to heal – (not if infection obvious).

DENDRITIC ULCER

The herpes simplex virus is a conjunctival commensal. Under a trigger such as stress or ultraviolet light it multiplies in the corneal epithelium breaking its surface, destroying its pain sensation and, if improperly treated, going on to produce a corneal scar infiltrated with blood vessels. The vessels ruin the corneal clarity but like all specialized tissues the cornea is prepared to sacrifice what makes it special in order to survive.

An allergic response to the virus (disciform keratitis) sometimes clouds the stroma with a disc-shaped opacity.

Examination

The branching figure whence the name is derived is neatly picked out in green with sodium fluorescein.

Figure 11.3
Keratitis. Dendritic ulcer. One of the three serious red eyes. Ciliary injection is not marked. The small dendritic figure is outlined in green with fluorescein

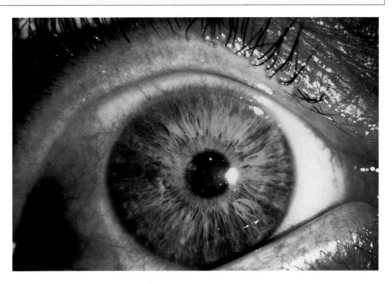

Action

The drug of choice today is acyclovir. Its selective toxicity inhibits virus replication without inhibiting replication of the host cell. It should be applied five times a day and continued for some days after healing is apparent.

Acyclovir has now eclipsed all of the other antivirals, and five times a day is not a tentative extension of the scriptural dosage of four times a day. It is at its most effective this way.

In the *long term*, tape closure of the eyelids is the most effective way to allow the corneal epithelium to regenerate because destruction of the corneal pain sensation has removed its only defence mechanism. Continued protection through artificial tears and occasional tape closure may help resist future herpetic outbreaks.

NB: The use of corticosteroids in the presence of an active dendritic ulcer amounts to malpractice.

BACTERIAL ULCER

Corneal laceration or perforation is a path or entry port for any pathogenic organism which happens to be in the vicinity. An abscess develops as a white fluffy opacity in the corneal stroma.

Action

In the *short term* start intensive topical antibiotics – usually chloramphenicol.

In the *longer term*, if scars develop following either viral or bacterial infection the only treatment may be a corneal graft. The cornea accepts the graft more happily than do other tissues because it has no blood vessels. Unfortunately, corneal ulcers may result in abnormal blood vessels that carry with them the antibodies of rejection.

CORNEAL EROSION

Patients complain of intense watering and pain on opening the eyelids, easing during the day and recurring at frequent and irregular intervals.

The corneal epithelium, dislodged from its connection with Bowman's membrane, adheres overnight to the eyelid instead, which on opening tears it away from the eye.

A history of the accident is found frequently in mothers gazing in admiration at their little bundles, from whom the last thing they expect is a punch in the eye.

Examination

The broken area is outlined with sodium fluorescein.

Action

No topical medication can make the corneal epithelium grow again. In the *short* term, tape closure is the only way to allow it to heal. In the *longer term*, however, once the epithelium has recovered some lubricants such as topical castor oil instilled nightly for up to 6 months will prevent the dreadful adhesion.

SATURDAY NIGHT EYE

When the festivities of an evening give way to deep slumber, the headache in the morning is further complicated by fierce pain when the eyes appear to open. The problem is that they have not been fully closed. Dehydration of the epithelium coupled with general dehydration causes exquisite agony when the capacity for sensation returns and the eyes open further still to discover what happened the night before.

Action

As for corneal erosion.

CORNEAL FOREIGN BODY

Presentation

- A sense of irritation on movement of the eyelid.
- A history of exposure to foreign material which may have been travelling fast enough to penetrate the globe.

Figure 11.4
Turning the upper lid. Traction applied to the lashes. A stick or glass rod pressing the upper edge of the tarsal plate backwards

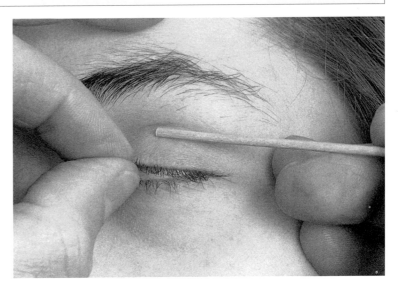

Figure 11.5
The conjunctiva. The upper lid exposed. Pressure on the lower lid paradoxically, brings the upper conjunctival fornix down over the cornea

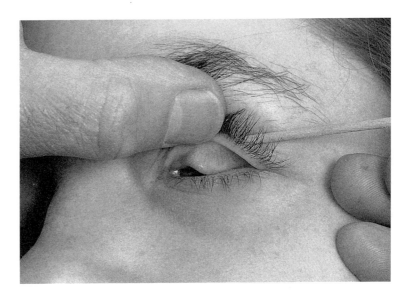

Grinding, drilling, hammering and chiselling without goggles are the classic start to such a history. There may be little evidence of any disaster to begin with.

Examination

Tiny fragments on the corneal surface can be seen with a small magnifying glass. Penetrating foreign bodies may not be seen at all. They must be diagnosed by the history and confirmed by radiograph.

Figure 11.6
Superficial corneal foreign bodies
are not uncommon. Removal should
be tried first with a cotton bud
under topical anaesthesia. A needle
may succeed when a cotton bud
fails

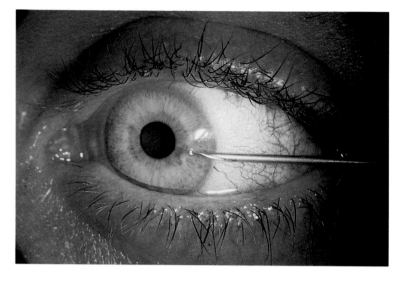

Action

Short term treatment comprises:

- Topical anaesthesia (amethocaine/benoxinate).
- Brush the fragments with a cotton tipped stick.
- If the stick fails, a 19 gauge needle will cause significantly less damage to the corneal epithelium than will the traditional corneal spud which might be better employed displayed in a museum.

If a penetrating injury is suspected then referral to an ophthalmic unit is obligatory.

CORNEAL LACERATION

Presentation

The history will be self-evident.
    The laceration is:

- a perfect entry portal for infection
- a perfect exit portal for ocular contents should any careless pressure be applied to the globe.

Whatever the patient might think, there may still be a retained intraocular foreign body which will eventually destroy the eye by infection, by the deposition of metallic salts throughout vital tissues or by fibrotic shrinkage of the retina or vitreous.

Action

Topical antibiotics and a pad are probably the safest first aid measure prior to referral to an ophthalmic unit.

IRITIS

A common condition, often with no adequate explanation, iritis has already been used as a model to demonstrate the ocular response to common pathology. Its effects on the eye in the acute phase differ markedly from those in the late fibrotic phase.

Figure 11.7
Acute iritis – one of the three serious red eyes. Usually presents with more pain than redness. Inflammatory adhesions may stick the iris to the lens where they are given the name of posterior synechiae

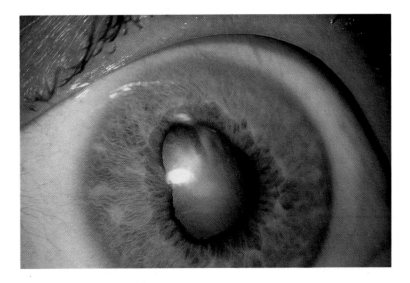

Presentation

The patient's complaint is often vague – a combination of:

- pain
- redness
- blurring of vision.

Examination

The external corneal surface is clear but deposits of inflammatory material (keratic precipitates), like flotsam and jetsam discarded by the sea, can be detected on the deep surface with a magnifying glass.

The pupil may be:

- spastic

Figure 11.8
Inflammatory debris on the deep
surface of the cornea (keratic
precipitates)

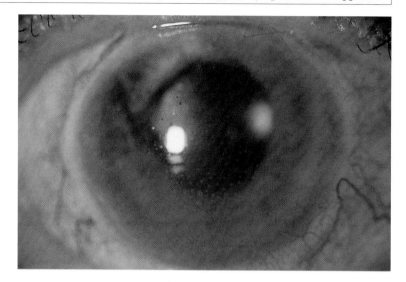

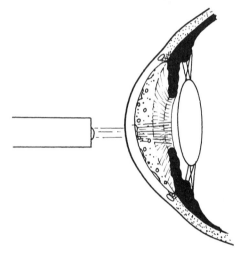

- distorted by previous adhesions
- dilated with atropine by the patient in anticipation of the same old treatment again.

Anterior chamber flare is a sign not easily picked up without a slit lamp.

Action

- Intensive topical corticosteroids to suppress the inflammation.
- Mydriatics (atropine or cyclopentolate) to relax the iris spasm and dilate the pupil.
- (a) systemic acetazolamide; (b) topical anti-glaucoma drops to combat any rise of intraocular pressure.

ACUTE ANGLE CLOSURE

Until the acute attack occurs the condition is not so much a disease as a shape – found in long-sighted, sometimes squinting eyes, which are too small internally for the safe dilatation of the pupil.

Presentation

- Intense headache and severely blurred vision.
- Through the patient's distress we may uncover a story of
  - (a) rainbow haloes
  - (b) frontal headaches
  - (c) transient attacks of blurred vision in the evening
  - (d) a spurious diagnosis of evening migraine.

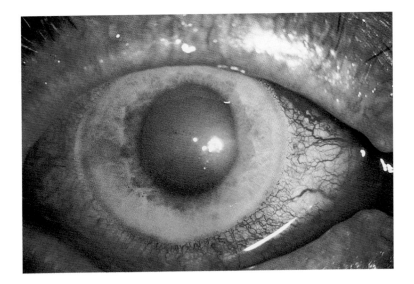

Figure 11.9
Acute angle closure – one of the three serious red eyes. Pupil fixed and dilated. The anterior chamber shallow. The pressure rock hard

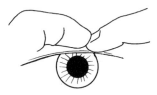

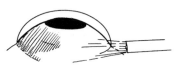

Examination

- The cornea is steamy and oedematous, sometimes obscuring the deeper signs.
- The pupil, if seen, will be fixed and dilated.
- The anterior chamber in both eyes is shallow. (If it is obscured on the affected side, an eclipse test on the fellow eye will leave the iris remote from the light in the shadow.)
- The eye will be rock hard and acutely tender.

Action

In the short term, the intraocular pressure must be reduced as a matter of some urgency.

- Systemic acetazolamide 500 mg immediately by vein or by mouth.
- Topical miotics – pilocarpine 2%
  (a) intensively to the affected eye
  (b) four times daily to the fellow eye to prevent pupil dilatation.

In the long term:

- Surgical peripheral iridectomies; or
- Yag laser iridotomies – both to bypass the pupillary block.
- An external drainage may be necessary if the trabecular meshwork has been damaged.

THE REASON WHY

It is commonly believed that acute angle closure is simply chronic simple glaucoma suddenly accelerating with pain and haloes. This is manifest nonsense. There is no connection between the two unless someone is unfortunate enough to have both.

The eye is long-sighted with an anterior chamber too shallow for safe dilatation. The advance of middle age exaggerates this shallowness, by forward movement of the iris and lens.

Extreme long sight has two further associates:

- thick convex glasses
- not infrequently, a convergent squint dating from childhood.

Passive dilatation of the pupil is not the whole story. Active dilatation under the influence of the sympathetic nervous system drags the iris back against the lens and blocks the pupil. It is for this reason that simple dilatation with, say, cyclopentolate does not always reveal patients at risk.

Like a character from a Greek tragedy, the eye appears to be at peace with its fatal flaw. Then the harbingers of doom issue their brief warnings. There are fleeting elevations of pressure. A swollen cornea breaks up the light into rainbow haloes and blurs the vision. Pain in the forehead can be mistaken for evening migraine and it is not unusual for patients to be subjected to extremes of neurological examination if the significance of the shallow anterior chamber is missed. The unities of drama do not need to be obeyed in real life.

The final disaster need not be inevitable. If we cannot always prove that someone is certainly going to have an acute attack of angle closure, at least we can identify those at risk, warn them what to expect and at least save them the anxiety of needless investigation by neurologists and ENT surgeons and the prescription of speculative treatment for conditions that they do not have.

12

Common disorders of the outer eye

The outer eye is an alliance – a coalition of partners linked together for their mutual benefit. Their association is not unlike that of the Common Market before it became the European Union.

Outside, we have Holland, represented by the eyelids, on the fringe, keeping danger out, protecting vital structures within. The conjunctiva, of course, is France – with her shadowy folds and tendency to become inflamed from time to time. The cornea, important, round, smooth – a transmitter of light – has to be Germany. Whilst Britain, all tearful nostalgia for when the world was young, can have no serious rivals as the lacrimal gland.

Figure 12.1
The alliance of the external eye: eyelids; conjunctiva; tears; cornea

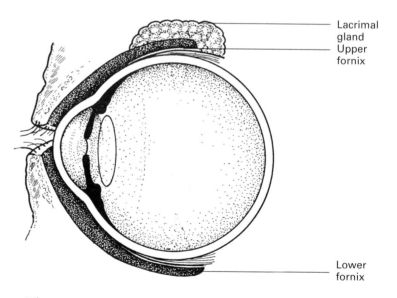

Lacrimal gland

Upper fornix

Lower fornix

The outer eye is a moist structure and, like the mouth, is most comfortable when shut. Also like the mouth, it has to open from time to time. Because of this, its entire arrangement allows the eye to experience, when open, the comfort it enjoys when shut – provided that it does not stay open for too long.

The cornea is protected by its pain sensation and the eyelashes, like cats' whiskers, trigger reflex closure of the lids when touched. In addition, the lids, continually blinking, spread tears over the cornea clearing away debris and producing optical perfection.

The conjunctival folds are not superfluous. They allow free movement of the eye and the conjunctival glands contribute fat and mucous to the tears. Without the conjunctiva and the tear glands there would be no eye.

Presentation

1 Extreme pain and discomfort on movement of the eyelids.
2 Watering and discharge.

CONJUNCTIVITIS

There can be no diagnosis more frequent than conjunctivitis even when it is actually something else. Any inflammation of the conjunctiva is conjunctivitis, secondary to whatever is near enough to be to blame – like a lacerated lid or irritation from a foreign body beneath the lid. The redness of conjunctivitis, whilst dominant and more dramatic than that of the major three, is not dominant around the corneoscleral limbus.

Figure 12.2
Acute conjunctivitis: normal cornea; normal pupil; normal anterior chamber; normal intraocular pressure (unless raised for other reasons)

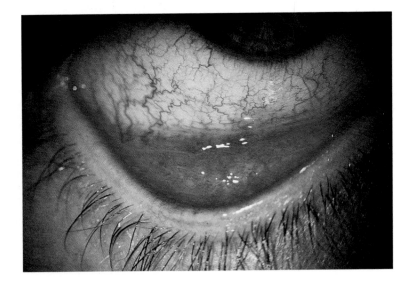

The causes are legion and infection need not be bacterial. Conducive factors are:

- lack of tears
- allergy
- chemical irritation
- radiation
- position of the eyelids (inwards or outwards)

Examination

The eye may be fiery and red and painful but:

- the *cornea* is lustrous and normal
- the *pupil* has no reason to be abnormal
- the *pressure* has no reason to be raised.

Action

Medical judgement should not be suspended because the eye looks fearful.

Short term management consists of:

- intensive topical antibiotics – chloramphenicol, gentamicin – should be applied every hour or even more often. Padding the eye actually hinders recovery. Viral conjunctivitis will take its own time – usually about 3 weeks – but antibiotics will limit a secondary infection.
- As a mark of perfection, culture should be taken of any discharge.

In the *long term* tear deficiency not only opens the door to infection it also irritates the eye in its own right. There are many artificial tear preparations. The gel based are more effective for longer. Cautery of the upper puncta sometimes obviates the need for any of them.

Presentation

The complaint is of sudden redness. Although usually described as painless, there is a slight dragging sensation. The vision is not affected.

SUBCONJUNCTIVAL HAEMORRHAGE

The sudden presence of blood scattered over a wide area of sclera can terrify both the patient and the doctor into a diagnosis of something dreadful.

Figure 12.3
Subconjunctival haemorrhage – of no consequence unless, rarely, a recurrent sign of a generalized bleeding tendency: normal vision; normal cornea; normal pupil; normal anterior chamber; normal intraocular pressure

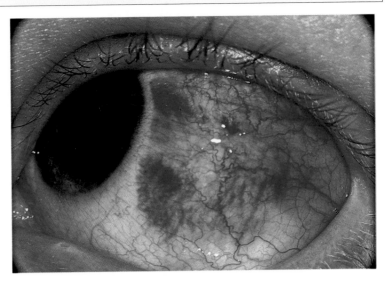

Figure 12.4
Subconjunctival haemorrhage – warfarin complicating minor surgery. A bulging conjunctiva is the tip of an iceberg of blood deep in the orbit, possibly blocking the vortex veins and raising the intraocular pressure

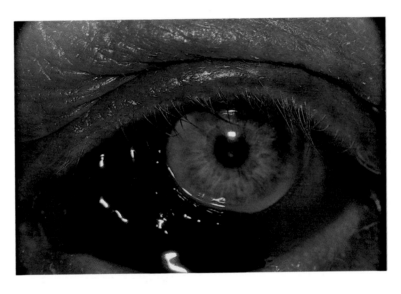

Examination

The seven markers are normal, in particular:

- the cornea
- the pupil
- the intraocular pressure (unless a gross orbital haemorrhage overflows into the conjunctiva)

but there is a total obliteration of the vascular markings.

Action

No treatment is necessary, but a subconjunctival haemorrhage is still a haemorrhage and has to be explained. Recurrent bouts of such bleeding require a routine search for a reason to bleed.

Presentation

Irritation on moving the eyelids.

CONCRETIONS

Concretions are tiny calcareous deposits in the tarsal conjunctiva. It is possible that epithelium folding on itself acts as an irritant, which the eye like an oyster rolls into a pearl. Sadly the pearl is not smooth and may in time fret against the corneal epithelium with predictable results.

Action

The concretions may be scraped away with a needle under topical anaesthesia.

Presentation

*   Swelling of the lid.
*   Intense pain.
*   The wrong assumption that the problem is a stye.

TARSAL CYST

When a stagnant tarsal gland becomes infected it turns into an abscess within the eyelid. When the infection fades away, the cyst hardens into a small lump (chalazion) which, if large enough, can distort vision.

Action

Short term: Intensive topical antibiotics usually bring about complete resolution and should be continued for some days after resolution appears to have occurred.

Long term: If resolution is incomplete, the cyst requires to be curetted from the deep surface of the lid.

Figure 12.5
Infected tarsal cyst – not beside a
lash root and therefore not a stye

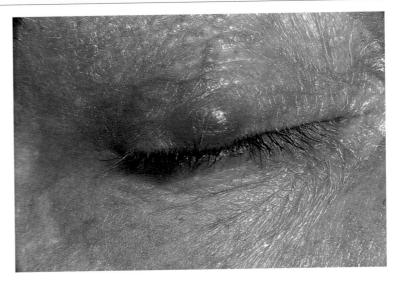

STYE (HORDEOLUM)

This is the diagnosis often applied to what generally turns
out to be a tarsal cyst. A true stye is infection of the lash
root and in the acute phase may be too painful to allow the
distinction to be made.

Action

Short term: The same as for infected tarsal cyst.
   Long term: Recurrent infections can be suggestive of some
underlying condition, such as diabetes.

Presentation

- Watering.
- Discharge.
- In children with asthma and eczema.

ATOPIC KERATO-CONJUNCTIVITIS

Fine papillae on the conjunctival surface of the lower eyelid
are the hallmark of a condition which is effectively conjunctival eczema. The papillae can abrade the corneal surface
into an ulcer.

Action

In the *short* term topical corticosteroids suppress the
conjunctival inflammation. The danger of corticosteroids

has to be balanced against that of the papillae. Once the epithelium is broken, a bandage contact lens keeps the papillae away from the healing corneal surface.

In the *long* term, sodium chromoglycate – happily without side effects and sometimes unhappily without any effect at all – may help prevent the development of these palpebral lesions. In time, as the asthma and eczema subside, so do the conjunctival papillae.

Presentation

The same watering and discharge as in the last condition but worse in the hay fever season.

SPRING CATARRH

Large papillae on the conjunctival surface of both upper and lower lids make corneal abrasions more likely than do the smaller papillae of atopic kerato-conjunctivitis.

Figure 12.6
Spring catarrh – giant papillae on the palpebral conjunctiva. The lid, instead of protecting the eye, works over it like a scrubbing brush

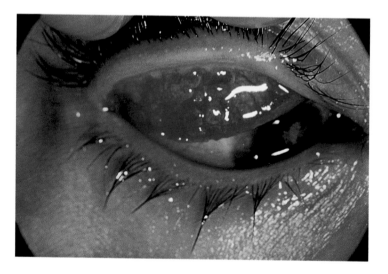

Action

Measures similar to those used in the previous condition.

Presentation

A painful inflammatory nodule, usually associated with nothing in particular. The nodule is heaped in one area.

EPISCLERITIS

Examination

The seven markers are normal, in particular:

- the cornea
- the pupil
- the intraocular pressure.

Inflammation is localized and elevated.

Action

Intensive topical corticosteroids, which may have to be repeated from time to time.

Presentation

- Pain and irritation in the eyes.
- Sporadic blotchy elevations over the face.

ROSACEA

Rosacea is a metabolic disturbance that produces blotchy inflammation over the cheeks and may also affect the eyes, producing the same blotchy inflammation in the conjunctiva and inflammatory opaque elevations across the cornea itself.

Scars in the cornea are the major danger, and new vessels with rejecting antibodies make a corneal graft unlikely to succeed.

Action

Short term: Topical corticosteroids suppress the acute phase.

Long term: Systemic tetracycline in a low dosage can prevent attacks altogether. A total ban on alcohol, spicy cuisine and other pleasing diversions has been recommended, but there is no record that colonial administrators sustained on a diet of burra pegs and fierce curries had a greater incidence of blotchy faces than did anyone else.

Presentation

- Pain.
- Later, crusting pustules form over the entire distribution of the ophthalmic division of the trigeminal nerve.

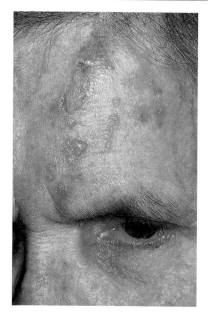

Figure 12.7
Shingles. The popular name for
herpes zoster ophthalmicus –
infection along the division of the
trigeminal nerve. Systemic acyclovir
has turned this full blown picture
into a rarity

SHINGLES (HERPES ZOSTER OPHTHALMICUS)

Infection is by the chicken pox virus (varicella). Vesicles change to pustules and form thick tenacious crusts, which appear in crops and sprays over the forehead and the upper eyelid.

This sequence of vesicle to pustule to scar affects:

- the skin – **dermatitis**
- the conjunctiva – **conjunctivitis**
- the cornea – **keratitis** (broken areas of corneal epithelium)
- the iris – **iritis**.

Examination

The distribution of lesions is so classic as to be diagnostic. Redness dominates around the corneoscleral limbus (keratitis).

- The corneal surface may be broken.
- The anterior chamber carries the aqueous flare of iritis.
- The intraocular pressure may be raised. (It could well be raised in the other eye also because we are now in the age group of chronic glaucoma.)

Action

Short term

- Topical antibiotics reduce the risk of secondary infection.
- Topical corticosteroids limit scar formation.
- Analgesics may relieve the pain. (Shingles most aptly has been called the girdle of roses from hell.)

Long term: The pain may continue for several months.

- Raised intraocular pressure may require permanent treatment.
- Cataract may require extraction.

Prevention

Acyclovir, which has had such dramatic success in the treatment of herpes simplex, can be equally effective for herpes zoster. Tablets at four times the standard dosage, 800 mg five times daily for 7 days, should be started before the vesicles become apparent. Such management might be thought to call for a degree of clairvoyance.

MALPOSITION OF THE EYELIDS

Wherever the lids turn – in or out – the lid margin is no longer in proper contact with the cornea and the alliance is broken.

Eyelid turning out (ectropion)

The same appearance may be produced in younger people by:

- a facial palsy
- contraction of a scar.

More serious is a laceration, tearing the margin and dropping the lid into two separate halves.

Figure 12.8
Ectropion. The cornea is exposed, the eye waters and the palpebral conjunctiva turns to skin

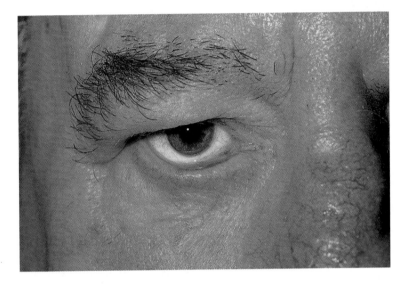

The danger of all is that of corneal exposure with:

- the drying conjunctiva turning to skin
- the drying cornea prepared to exchange clarity for survival.

Presentation

Watering and discomfort (although surprisingly, not always).

Examination

- The lid no longer contacts the eye.
- The conjunctiva becomes keratinized.

- The exposed cornea may develop punctate erosions (staining with fluorescein).
- There may be frank bacterial infection.

Action

We must:

- deal with the consequences of exposure
- reverse the exposure.

Short term measures:

- Topical lubrication to reduce loss of moisture from evaporation with
  (a) artificial tears
  (b) simple white paraffin ointment.
- Closing the lids with adhesive tape certainly puts an end to exposure but the eyes see better when open.

Long term action:

- Removal of a wedge from the lower lid to pull the margin back against the eyeball.
- Relief of cicatricial contraction.
- Repair of any laceration – all with special care to restore the integrity of the lid margin.

Eyelid turning in (entropion)
Connective tissue failure allows the eyelashes and skin to act independently when the underlying muscles contract. The lashes then work against the corneal epithelium like a scrubbing brush producing:

- excoriation of the corneal surface
- actual corneal infection.

Figure 12.9
Entropion. The lower lid turns inwards, abrading the corneal surface with the eyelashes

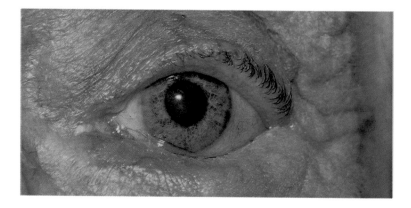

> **Presentation**
>
> Irritation of the eyes, particularly when the lids close tightly.

Action

Adhesive tape applied below the line of lashes can turn them away safely in the *short term*. In the *long term*, the cure is surgical, requiring either:

- stitches through the eyelids (Snellen's), or
- a more complicated wedge resection.

> **Presentation**
>
> Constant sense of irritation improved by lifting the lid from the eye.

TRICHIASIS

Aberrant lashes can produce the same complaints and effects as entropion without actual distortion of the eyelid.

Action

Ocular lubricants can protect the cornea in the short term. The lash roots can be destroyed with cryocoagulation or electrolysis for long term prevention.

> **Presentation**
>
> - Irritation.
> - Formation of scales and flakes around the roots of the eyelashes.

BLEPHARITIS

In its simple form this is essentially dandruff of the eyelashes. A more serious ulcerative form brings with it a destructive inflammation involving the adjacent skin as well.

Action

- The flecks that cluster round the base of the lashes have to be washed away with warm water.

- An antibiotic ointment such as chloramphenicol must be rubbed deeply into the lash roots, three or four times a day for three or four days at a time.

When the scales return, the whole process has to start again.

Presentation

Dryness and irritation of the eyes aggravated by central heating.

DRY EYE

Without tears the eye cannot exist. Reduced production of tears is not uncommon and exposes the eye to recurrent infections and punctate erosions of the cornea.

Action

In the *short term*, artificial tears, either a liquid or gel, can prolong the wetting time of the normal tear film.

A more radical *long term* approach is to block one of the outflow canaliculi. Since we have abandoned walking on all fours the upper canaliculus plays a less important role than it does in some monkeys. This duct, carrying away some 20% of the tears, can be blocked permanently with cautery. In cases of great severity, the lower punctum may be blocked also.

Presentation

The patient has observed a fleshy lump at the nasal corneo-scleral margin. There is always the unspoken fear that it might be a tumour.

PTERYGIUM

An accumulation of degenerative tissue deep to the nasal conjunctiva creeps across the cornea in the line of the opening eyelids dragging the conjunctiva with it in the form of a wing, hence its name. It may advance relentlessly across the cornea from one side to the other, trailing a scar over the pupil. Salt and wind at sea, icy blasts on the ski slopes and constant battering from sand make the condition more

Figure 12.10
Pterygium. Once the corneo-scleral
frontier is crossed, the corneal tissue
affected will forever be opaque.
Removal can only prevent further
opacity

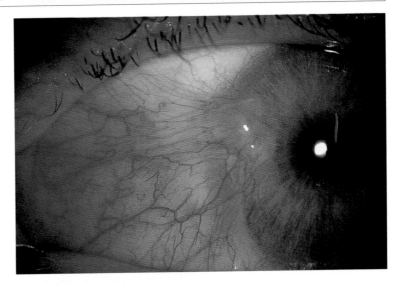

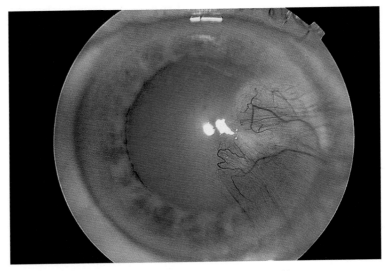

common in sailors, mountain sportsmen and desert Arabs. The condition is benign until it threatens to move across the cornea.

Pterygium is evident in the portraits of Admiral Nelson, the posthumous victor of Trafalgar classically celebrated as having lost an eye in endless battles with the French. In fact he had not. Contrary to popular belief he never wore a black patch and it is conceivable that he had not mentioned any visual improvement to the Admiralty for fear of losing his pension. A combination of presbyopia and pterygium is less heroic but likely to have done more harm to both eyes than did the French guns to one. There was still time for heroism during the surgical excisions without anaesthesia.

Action

If the cornea is not threatened, then inactivity on the part of the surgeon may be proved the best decision by equal inactivity on the part of the pterygium.

If the cornea is threatened, then excision must be attempted. The wide range of surgical options attests the failure to guarantee a cure every time.

NB: *The condition must not be confused with a pinguecula – a flabby yellow nodule that occupies the same area on the conjunctiva but never crosses on to the corneo-scleral frontier.*

THE ALLERGIC RESPONSE

Unfortunately all drugs, even those used to treat allergy have a capacity to provoke some allergic reaction themselves. In the eye, they are recognized by swelling of the tarsal conjunctiva and skin, with oedema spreading from the lid margin to beyond the orbital limits. In time, the skin takes on a leathery sheen, giving way to superficial flaking.

Action

Topical hydrocortisone is marvellously effective, but stopping the offending application is obligatory.

Figure 12.11
Topical medications share a common feature – their capacity to provoke an allergic inflammation (one-response organ)

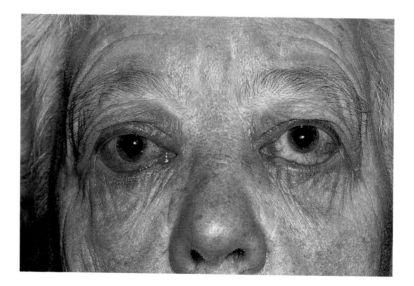

13

Glaucoma

The word glaucoma has about six different meanings, which we use interchangeably. To make matters worse, the word 'glaucous' still current in English, derives from the descriptions in early Greek medicine of eyes that were green, not with envy but with cataract.

Whilst today glaucoma certainly does not mean cataract, it can mean any one of the following:

- A pathological process (the best meaning).
- Any casual rise in intraocular pressure.
- Any pressure rise for which some agency has been identified (or not identified).
- The named disease – chronic simple glaucoma.
- The named disease – acute glaucoma (angle closure).
- The named disease – infantile glaucoma.

Presenting features
Most patients do not realize they have chronic glaucoma because a quiet rise in intraocular pressure and creeping field loss are not noticed. The condition is therefore without symptoms and, given the six different meanings, it is highly unlikely that anyone would have any idea which one they should be suspecting.

CHRONIC SIMPLE GLAUCOMA

Glaucoma simplex is the name given to that neuropathy of the optic nerve which, untreated, leads on to glaucoma the pathological process, whose characteristics may safely tolerate repetition.

- Defects within the visual field (arcuate scotoma), leading on to loss of contour on the nasal side, detectable with the hands.

- In most cases an intraocular pressure that fluctuates throughout the day above 20 mmHg.
- Extension of the normal round optic cup into a vertical oval.

Figure 13.1
Chronic glaucoma: cupped disc; field loss; raised intraocular pressure

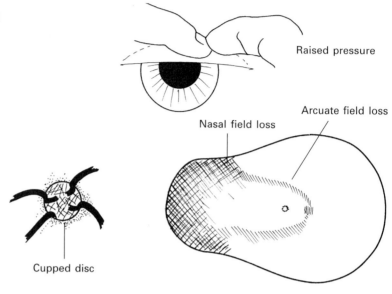

Raised pressure

Arcuate field loss

Nasal field loss

Cupped disc

NB: Chronic glaucoma with its normal anterior chamber is not an idle version of acute glaucoma. Such eyes will tolerate a dilated pupil and hence will tolerate all those pupil-dilating drugs banned in the formularies for use in patients with 'glaucoma'. Pupil-dilating drugs are dangerous only when angle closure is threatened.

Pathology

The 'simple' in the name is a medical codeword for complex. The cause is not known although it is assumed that the trabecular meshwork, for whatever reason, does not function properly. Because the optic nerve is also ischaemic, its blood flow can be dangerously compromised by even a mild pressure rise.

Action

If everybody over the age of 40 acquired the habit of having the eyes checked every 2 years by an optician, then everybody with chronic simple glaucoma would be detected in time to prevent needless damage. It is remarkable how many people still believe the disease to be untreatable yet the tragedy is not to have it but not to know one has it until it is too late.

Despite the existence of a certain percentage of people whose field loss and cupped discs are associated with a normal intraocular pressure, the medical aim is to reduce the intraocular pressure to a level at which the field loss is arrested. Such treatment takes the form of:

- topical medication – usually
- oral treatment – occasionally
- argon laser trabeculoplasty – occasionally, where a series of laser burns appears to improve trabecular efficiency
- surgical drainage.

Beta adrenergic antagonists

There are four main drugs which decrease aqueous flow:

- timolol
- carteolol
- betaxolol
- levobunolol.

All beta blockers can:

- produce bronchospasm, and
- slow the pulse rate to dangerous levels, particularly in the presence of cardiac failure.

Even in people with no recognized cardiopulmonary disease, a reduced cardiac output reduces their capacity to exercise. There is also the problem of vasospasm in cold extremities which raises the possibility of the same vasospasm in a 'cold' optic nerve.

They are generally used twice daily.

Cholinergics

Pilocarpine, with its 100-year track record, is still prescribed. It probably increases the outflow at the trabecular meshwork but its side effects are even more marked than those of the beta blockers.

Although it is very effective, the price paid is extreme meiosis, which darkens the vision and makes patients wonder why the glaucoma clinic staff are so delighted with their management of a condition that was without visual loss before treatment was started. It induces myopia in young patients, and long term, it militates against successful drainage surgery and hinders pupil dilatation.

Because new formulations have come into vogue, pilocarpine in chronic glaucoma should now be sliding into the pages of history.

Sympathomimetics

Adrenalin—Adrenalin and its pro-drug formulation may in certain patients increase outflow through the trabecular meshwork and through the sclera, but like pilocarpine, they are becoming of historical interest only.

Alpha-agonists

Brimonidine—Although likely to produce ocular irritation, it is as effective as timolol in reducing intraocular pressure and may well become in the future a first line alternative to beta blockers. It reduces the aqueous inflow and increases the uveo-scleral outflow.

Carbonic anhydrase inhibitors

Acetazolamide—This drug (like its relation, dichlorphenamide) reduces aqueous production. Oral treatment can only have a short term role when rapid reduction of intraocular pressure is called for. Its long term side effects make continued use unacceptable. All patients will experience tingling of the extremities whilst a significant majority will complain of lethargy, digestive disorders and occasionally suffer renal calculi.

Dorzolamide—This is the first carbonic anhydrase inhibitor capable of lowering the intraocular pressure when delivered topically. It can be used three times daily in addition to beta blockers but the likelihood of allergy and the unpleasant taste experienced during usage might militate against its general acceptance.

Latanoprost—This topical prostaglandin on a once daily basis would appear to lower the intraocular pressure more effectively than timolol. It increases the uveo-scleral outflow and may well open a new chapter in the management of raised intraocular pressure.

Predictably, any drug with good effects can have bad effects. Latanoprost can induce redness and may increase iris pigmentation.

Surgery

The present favoured operation (trabeculectomy) substitutes a small hole in the trabecular meshwork allowing the free passage of aqueous from the anterior chamber eventually into the subconjunctival space. The size of the hole has to be just right, because one too small will not drain and one too big will drain too much. The first leaves us very much where we were to begin with, the second results in:

- a soft eye
- a flattened anterior chamber, and
- eventual cataract, resulting from upset aqueous dynamics.

A laser-induced drainage channel may soon turn these complications into the difficulties of yesterday.

14

The cranial nerves

When patients present primarily with a disorder of the eye, there is usually neither time nor space to carry out a full neurological examination. In addition, there is rarely any point, because the neurologists do it better and if we have felt moved to try it ourselves, we probably suspect something that is going to be referred to them anyway.

Some ophthalmic conditions, however, give a hint of a neurological component although there are no symptoms directly referable to the central nervous system.

Figure 14.1
The cranial nerves, near companions at their source, tend to separate as they leave the brain stem

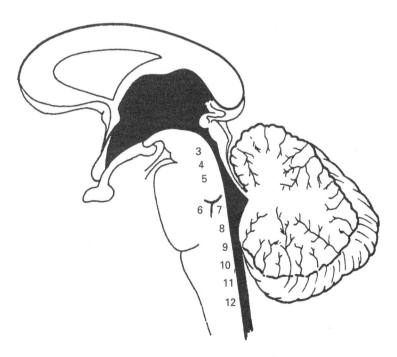

The cranial nerves are readily accessible without the need for a couch or a chaperone. If they are intact, it is highly likely that the central nervous system is intact also. Nor should it be forgotten that the second, third, fourth, fifth, sixth and seventh nerves all influence the eyes in one way or another.

In certain cases, a radiograph of the skull – or as modern technology demands, a CT or MRI scan –.might give information on the following points.

- A large pituitary fossa usually indicates a large gland and a large gland can compress the visual pathways into field defects in optic atrophy which may mimic the appearances of chronic glaucoma.
- Abnormal calcification sometimes outlines the wall of a carotid aneurysm or disperses within the substance of a tumour.
- Disturbance like hyperostosis of intracranial bone could indicate a meningioma or some less common growth.

It would seem to be a universal experience in every medical school that instruction tends to come to a halt with the teacher's departure for lunch somewhere between the seventh and the eighth cranial nerve. This section is therefore designed for all of us who missed the last five and would like to be reminded about the first seven.

Olfactory

It has become customary to bypass the first nerve with a question or two about the sense of smell because the recommended wintergreen or oil of cloves has generally vanished.

Optic

The optic nerve, like the olfactory, is anatomically part of the brain. Two aspects of its function are tested routinely:

- vision
    (i) central
    (ii) field
- the pupil – light and accommodation.

Briskness of response and equality are the two prime features that indicate normality.

At this point in a textbook of ophthalmology neither should vision nor pupils require to be discussed further.

Although not strictly chronological, it makes sense to take the third, fourth and sixth cranial nerves together because the structures they innervate also work together.

Oculomotor

The third nerve has three functions:

- Its parasympathetic fibres form the outflow for the pupil reflex.

- Its motor fibres innervate the levator of the upper lid, and
- The movements of the eye in all directions except those supplied by the fourth and sixth nerves.

Trochlear

The superior oblique, innervated by the fourth nerve rotates the eye downwards *when it is in adduction*. Because adduction is impossible in the presence of a third nerve palsy, the oblique will instead rotate the upper surface of the eye towards the nose (intorsion). This sign is very subtle, much beloved by crusty examiners and probably of little use except to answer their questions.

Figure 14.2
The superior oblique (trochlear nerve) depresses the eye when it is turned inwards. If the eye cannot turn inwards (adduction), the superior oblique cannot depress it, in which case it rotates the eye downward to the nose (intorsion)

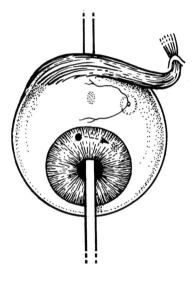

Abducent

The sixth cranial nerve innervates the lateral rectus.

The test (for all three)

- Can the upper lid be elevated?
- The pupil light reflex.
- The extraocular movements – *one eye at a time*.

Third nerve

A palsy will result in:

- a dropped upper lid (ptosis)
- a dilated pupil
- paralysis of all eye movements except that of
  the superior oblique – intorsion
  the lateral rectus nerve – abduction.

Figure 14.3
Right third nerve palsy: dropped
eyelid; dilated pupil; intact abduction
(lateral rectus)

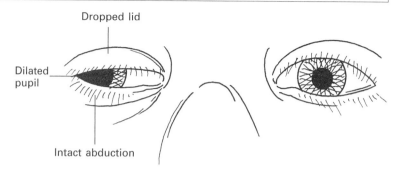

The eye will be abducted.

Fourth nerve
An isolated superior oblique palsy is rare.

The test

The order to look down is not followed by a downward movement of the adducted eye.

Sixth nerve
An isolated lateral rectus palsy on the other hand is very common.

The test

Limitation of the eye in abduction (outwards) – end point nystagmus.

Trigeminal
The fifth cranial nerve supplies sensation to the face in three great branches – ophthalmic, maxillary and mandibular – from the forehead to the temples and temples to the lower jaw. Not surprisingly, the first division supplies the sensation to the eye. Less obvious structures include the sinuses, all the contents of the mouth and the hard palate excluding:

• the posterior third of the tongue
• the soft palate.

It supplies the muscles of mastication.

The tests

• Sensory—Compare the right and left sensation to touch along the areas supplied by the three divisions:
  the temples (not forgetting the cornea)

Figure 14.4
The fifth nerve supplies sensation to the temples, cheeks and chin as well as the cornea and buccal mucous membranes. The muscles of mastication are served by the motor root

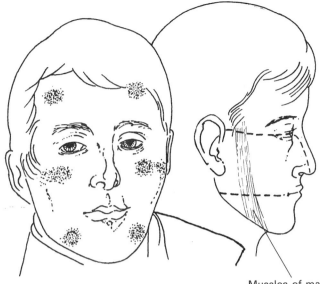

Muscles of mastication

the cheeks
the chin.
- **Motor**—Feel the masseters when the teeth are clenched.

Facial
The seventh nerve is mainly motor to the muscles of facial expression. It also supplies parasympathetic:

- secretory fibres to the lacrimal gland
- taste fibres to the anterior two thirds of the tongue.

The tests

Motor—The unaffected muscle pulls the paralysed face towards the unaffected side. Because the muscles of the forehead have bilateral representation in the motor cortex, an *upper motor neurone palsy* will leave the whole forehead *wrinkling equally*.

Bilateral representation is irrelevant in a *lower motor neurone palsy*, which paralyses the entire side of the face, including the forehead, leaving it immobile, unwrinkled and expressionless.

We should therefore:

- observe the direction of the dragging muscle.
- ask the patient to
  (a) wrinkle the forehead
  (b) squeeze the eyelids shut
  (c) blow through the lips as if to whistle

Forehead smooth, therefore lower motor neurone lesion

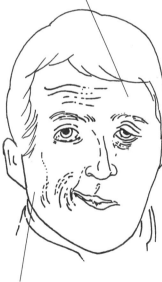

Normal side

Figure 14.5
Left facial palsy (lower motor neurone). The unaffected side pulls the weakened side towards it. An upper motor neurone lesion would have left the forehead wrinkling equal and intact

The eyelids fail to shut properly and the flaccid cheek and lip blow out towards the affected side.

Sensory—In theory we should offer for consideration:

- sugar – sweet
- citric acid – sour
- quinine – bitter
- salt (obvious) – in this order.

As ever, the necessary materials are not usually to hand.

Acoustic
The eighth nerve serves both hearing and balance.

The tests

Hearing—A light noise is presented to each ear. The practice of whispering inanities into just one ear then the other could well be regarded as suggestive. Less provocative is the forefinger fretting against the thumb, which requires no equipment. Since few of us carry timepieces with audible ticks this tradition has slipped into history. If genuine deafness be discovered, we may proceed to the tuning fork. The names Rinne and Weber were probably the last eponyms cast forth before the teacher disappeared for lunch. Whilst it is comforting to know that fragments of youth can still be prised from the depths of an ageing memory, practical principles are more likely to lurk near the surface ready for action without the added burden of yet another name.

Figure 14.6
The tuning fork test. Air conduction of sound is better than bone conduction in the absence of middle ear disease. Neither air nor bone conduction can overcome nerve deafness

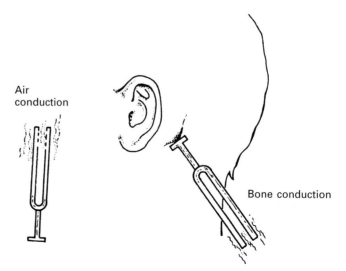

Air conduction

Bone conduction

Conduction of noise through air is better than through bone – *provided the middle ear is intact*. A vibrating fork is placed on the mastoid until it is heard no more then it is placed by the open ear.

- A normal ear will hear it.
- An ear with middle ear disease will not.
- An ear with nerve deafness will not hear it at all – through bone or air.

Balance—Changing position of the head in this way produces fluid movements within the semi-circular canals. If the head is then held static, a circling flow of fluid will make the eyes move instead – *provided the vestibular apparatus is normal*. Such movement can be induced by changing the temperature adjacent to the canals by pouring either hot or cold water into the external ear. The resultant nystagmus will twitch one way for hot, the other for cold. The respective directions are remembered only by neurologists and sometimes by examination candidates.

Glossopharyngeal
The ninth nerve:

- innervates movements of the soft palate
- supplies sensation to
    (a) the pharynx and its neighbours, and
    (b) the sense of taste to the posterior third of the tongue.

The tests

When the patient says 'aah' –

- The pharynx *in health* constricts, raising the uvula in the centre line.
- *In disease*, the uvula is moved to the normal side as does the face in seventh nerve palsy.

Paralysed side

Figure 14.7
The response to the request to say 'aah' arches the healthy palate but fails to arch the side supplied by a non-functioning glossopharyngeal and vagus nerve. As with a seventh nerve palsy, the weak side is dragged towards the strong side

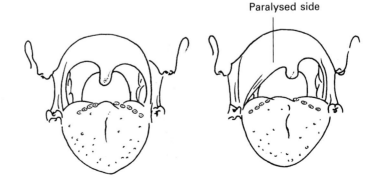

Many patients, particularly those who have not understood the aim of the cranial nerve examination feel that being asked to do this test is to put them at a moral disadvantage especially if their tongue is more coated than they would like to be thought normal for them.

The gag reflex—Anyone who has been examined by an ear, nose and throat surgeon would not willingly inflict this on anybody else, and to push it further by testing for taste is not likely to be successful. A patient who is about to vomit will not be in a position to distinguish between sweet, sour, bitter or salt.

Vagus

The tenth nerve serves many purposes, but in essence:

- It joins the ninth in movements of the soft palate.
- It innervates the extrinsic muscles of the larynx.
- It slows the heart.
- It excites gut movement and secretion.

The tests

Although clearly wandering further than the ninth nerve as its name applies, only the functions shared with the ninth nerve can be tested in a consulting room.

Accessory

The eleventh nerve joins the tenth as the tenth joins the ninth, and its main role is to innervate the trapezius and the sterno-mastoid muscles.

Figure 14.8
Pressure of the hand against the resisting head tests for an intact accessory nerve

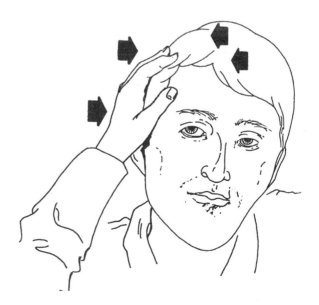

The tests

The muscles can be brought into action by:

- shrugging the shoulders
- rotating the head against resistance.

Hypoglossal
The twelfth nerve supplies the muscles of the tongue.

The tests

During the act of sticking out the tongue, the healthy side pushes the tongue towards the affected side. This is quite the opposite to what happens with paralysis of the:

- facial nerve
- glossopharyngeal nerve.

Figure 14.9
Hypoglossal palsy. The tongue is pushed towards the damaged side. This is in direct contrast to paralysis of the seventh, ninth and tenth nerves

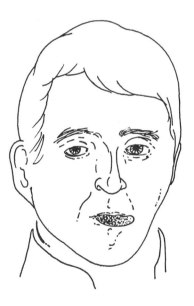

INTRACRANIAL DISORDERS

Intracranial tumours
The eyes, as the external representatives of the brain, can be affected in several ways by lesions that take up space within the unyielding confines of the skull.

Raised intracranial pressure
- Headaches, worse in the morning and easing by gravity when the recumbent position is abandoned, must always

be taken seriously, particularly if the headaches progress relentlessly.

- The long intracranial pathway of the sixth nerve makes it vulnerable in a non-locating way to rising intracranial pressure.
- A swollen optic nerve head (without visual loss) is regarded as a classic associate.

Ocular motility
Eye movements can be affected in two ways, either by:

- frank paralysis of the muscles supplied by the third (including the pupil), fourth and sixth cranial nerves, and
- nystagmus, usually brought about by tumours in the posterior fossa.

Visual disturbance
Positive—Disturbance of the temporal and parietal cortex particularly can give rise to formed hallucinations.

Negative—Field defects can occur from damage anywhere along the visual pathways. In particular those around the pituitary fossa may simulate the field defects of chronic simple glaucoma but without a raised pressure. We must not label anybody as having low tension glaucoma before first eliminating the possibility of an enlarged pituitary gland.

Altered appearance
Tumours, particularly a meningioma of the sphenoidal ridge, can displace the eye forwards. A facial nerve palsy, classically the result of an acoustic neuroma, inhibits lacrimal secretion but induces watering due to defective closure of the lower lid.

15

Nystagmus

Nystagmus for most doctors is a constant reminder that they should have paid more attention as students It is also possible that the cranial nerve instructor who disappeared at the eighth nerve may have intended to teach it after the twelfth.

The definition is simple enough: an involuntary repetitive oscillation of one or both eyes in any direction at any speed, and at any frequency.

It occurs when some lesion induces a malfunction in the normal mechanisms that initiate or modify eye movements. It is almost a parody of normality with defects that range across:

- ocular fixation
- paralysis of the extraocular movements
- dysfunction in
  - (a) the brain stem
  - (b) the cerebellum
  - (c) the vestibular apparatus.

Figure 15.1
The elements which control voluntary and involuntary eye movements. Nystagmus is a parody of normality resulting from: defects in ocular fixation; paralysis of extraocular movement; malfunction of the brain stem, cerebellum and vestibular apparatus

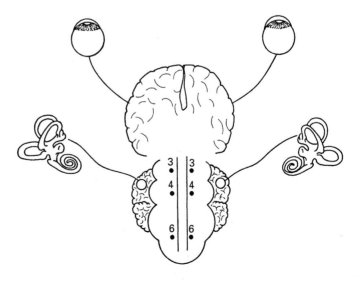

All these are linked to the eye movements through the nuclei of the third, fourth and sixth cranial nerves. They are under the influence of:

- Vision – unless it is defective for some reason or other.
- The otoliths, which give information about the *position* of the head in space.
- The semicircular canals which supply information about *movements* of the head in space.
- The cerebellum, which via the vestibular nucleii, imposes a fine restraint on the natural coarseness of eye movements.

The cause of nystagmus must therefore lie either in the eye or in the brain. Since most of the controlling elements lie in the brain then most of the causes for nystagmus must lie there also. They are not always found. All eyes with nystagmus move. That they move is almost invariably more important than how they move, except in two circumstances.

- Children whose eyes cannot fix have no mechanism for holding the eyes still in any position of gaze. They therefore develop searching movement for a point of rest that forever eludes them. Amplitude and speed are equal in both directions.
- End point nystagmus. General fatigue, and other weakening disorders make it difficult for the eyes to be held in extremes of lateral gaze. They drift back to the centre and are corrected by movement which takes the eyes rapidly back to the lateral position, whence the inward drift begins again.
- When the eyes move to the other side, the direction of the fast movement changes to that of the new direction of gaze.

NB: The end point drift occurs only in lateral gaze and never in the straight forward position. Occurring in one eye, it may be the first sign of a frank sixth nerve palsy.

Figure 15.2
End point nystagmus, the most common. The fast component beating to the right in dextroversion and the left in laevoversion means: exhaustion; debility; intoxication. To one side only could mean a partial sixth nerve palsy. The movements must be taken to the limits else the end point will not be reached

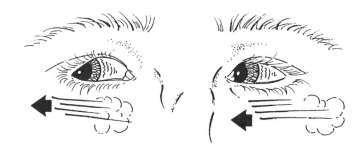

Latent nystagmus
This is really ocular nystagmus affecting one eye only when the dominant eye is covered.

Nystagmus of recent onset
In most circumstances, an abundance of other signs makes the discovery of nystagmus merely an interesting observation. Occasionally, however, it may be the presenting feature.

Ataxic
Some disturbance of the medial longitudinal bundle, usually demyelination, has an asymmetric effect on each eye:

- one fails to adduct
- the other fails to remain still.

Cerebellar
The cerebellum is the great coordinator: it does not initiate actions, it smoothes them. In its absence, the eyes jerk coarsely, as do muscles everywhere else in the body.

Posterior fossa tumour
Cerebellar jerks may be the first sign of a tumour in children who are symptomless in all other ways. It must be distinguished from ocular and latent nystagmus where the movements are equal and the eyes do not jerk.

Spasmus nutans
Very occasionally a 6-month-old baby embarks on a strange course of apparently pointless head nodding whilst jerking the eyes around in an asymmetric and equally pointless way. Since so much else in one's behaviour at 6 months old may appear pointless, it is wiser to regard this habit as of no consequence. The affected child will happily return to normality within a few more months, before investigation has put this likelihood at risk.

Summary
That the eyes move is more important than how they move.
  Nystagmus of recent origin requires to be explained:

- the brain stem – demyelination
- the cerebellum – usually tumour.

16

The pupil reflexes and some common pupil abnormalities

All reflexes behave in the same two ways:

- There is a neuromuscular response to stimulus.
- There is an inflow pathway and an outflow pathway.

THE PUPILS

The response is constriction only. The outflow is the third cranial nerve arising at the level of the mid-brain.

Figure 16.1
Normal pupils without and with light stimulation. Light on one constricts both – direct reflex and consensual reflex

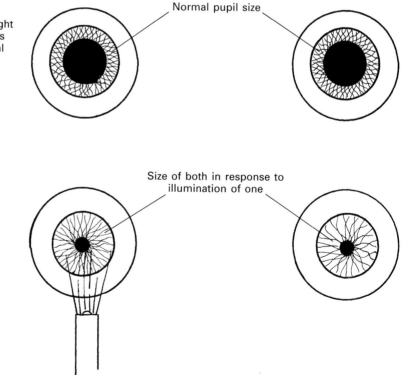

The stimulus is two-fold:

- *Light* (a strong torch must be used). Light travels by the retina and the optic nerve to the mid-brain.
- Focusing for near (*accommodation*): the pathway, although still controversial, is possibly initiated by the contraction of the medial rectus. It is nothing to do with actual vision because it can happen in a blind person asked to look towards the nose.

NB: Any blinding lesion behind the mid-brain – for example in the occipital cortex – has no influence on the pupil reflexes. In cases of cortical blindness, the pupil responses to light will be normal.

Because the nasal fibres in each retina cross at the chiasma it will cause both pupils to constrict:

- in the eye illuminated – the direct response
- in the fellow eye – the consensual response.

The direct response in health is always stronger than the consensual.

THE SWINGING LIGHT TEST

Normal response
- Light directed at the left eye will produce constriction of both pupils.
- When light is taken from the left to the right eye the pupils begin to dilate. When the light arrives, the right pupil constricts again.

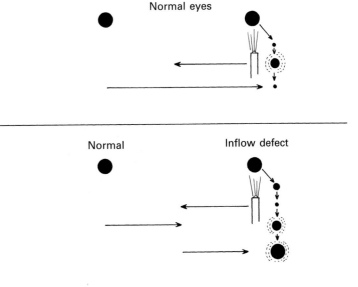

Figure 16.2
The swinging light test to reveal inflow defect: partial direct response from the first pupil; normal direct response from the second pupil; continued dilatation of the first pupil when the light shines on it again

Abnormal response

Inflow defects
Absolute defect—Such occurs when a central retinal artery occlusion has totally eliminated light perception. In such circumstances, light directed at the *affected eye* produces no constriction.

Relative afferent pupil defect RAPD
When visual loss is not total, as in a central retinal vein occlusion or optic neuritis, then the direct response in the affected eye will be weaker than the consensual.

Figure 16.3
Inflow defect. Light presented to the healthy eye constricts both. Light presented to the affected eye constricts neither

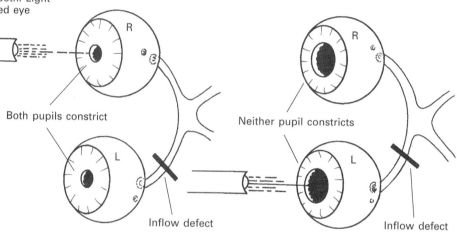

Both pupils constrict

Neither pupil constricts

Inflow defect

Inflow defect

- The *affected eye* will have a poorly sustained response to light (direct).
- The *fellow eye* will have a poorly sustained response (consensual).

When the torch is moved to the *unaffected eye*, both direct and consensual reflexes are brisk. By the time the light is swung back to the *first eye*, the pupil will have begun to dilate and despite the arrival of light, *it will dilate further still*.

Outflow defect
The affected eye will demonstrate:

- no direct reflex
- no consensual reflex.

Figure 16.4
Outflow defect. Light presented to the affected eye constricts only the pupil in the normal side. Light presented to the normal eye still constricts the same pupil

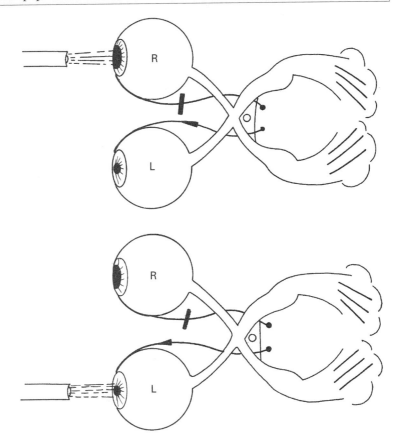

COMMON PUPIL ABNORMALITIES

Unequal but with normal light reactions

Such anisocoria may be normal for that person – a conviction confirmed by:

- absence of symptoms
- no positive findings in the ophthalmic ritual
- no positive findings in the cranial nerve examination.

The continued suspicion that one of the pupils is abnormal can be allayed or confirmed by carrying out the test in reduced illumination, when:

- the normal pupil will dilate further and then respond briskly to light, and
- the abnormal pupil will not dilate at all.

If both dilate equally then they are probably normal.

Dilated with sluggish or absent light reflexes – direct and consensual

The Holmes–Adie or tonic pupil is by tradition linked with absent knee jerk reflexes – an association that will not cause as much concern to the patient as will the failure of near focus. If the eye can still focus for near, the pupil will constrict eventually. The constriction and subsequent dilatation will be remarkably slow.

Chemical test—A weak (0.1%) solution of pilocarpine – the concentration that would have no effect on the normal eye – constricts the pupil in an affected eye because of denervation hypersensitivity.

Action

Reassurance, following a brisk passage through:

- the ophthalmic ritual
- the cranial nerves.

Dilated and fixed

Drug induced
Inadvertent installation of a mydriatic, for example atropine, is commoner than might be imagined.

Trauma
Traumatic mydriasis, although in itself not dangerous, follows a severe blow to the eye, which may have been severe enough to cause:

- damage to the drainage angle with a resultant secondary rise of pressure, *often years later*
- dislocation of the lens or cataract
- detachment of the retina due to a peripheral traumatic tear – *also months and years later.*

Dilated and fixed with other symptoms
In serious conditions like acute angle closure or a third nerve palsy, the dilated pupil is merely an incidental finding amongst other more commanding signs.

Small
Paralysis of the cervical sympathetic denervates the dilator pupillae of the affected side (Horner's syndrome) allowing:

- the pupil to shrink, and
- the upper lid to droop.

Action

Consideration must be given to:

- The ophthalmic ritual.
- The cranial nerves.
- We must always think of a mass at the thoracic outlet.

Small and fixed

Drug induced
Instillation of miotic drops (pilocarpine) is just as common as is the instillation of atropine.

The Argyll–Robertson pupil
The size should avoid confusion with the Holmes–Adie pupil. The old crammer's mnemonic was to liken the pupil to a student's garret of olden times as having 'accommodation but no light'.

The arrival of AIDS has now reduced syphilis to an obscure footnote in history, recalled only by gold medallists with the fanciful reminder that every admiral was once a midshipman and every bishop a divinity student.

Other small pupils
In pontine haemorrhage and opiate poisoning it is customary to describe the pupils as pinpoint, as indeed they are. However, there are other features which demand more attention.

Not all abnormal pupils have abnormal reflexes. Local conditions can alter the regular round appearance even though the reflex pathways are still intact. Injury, either accidental or surgical, can leave gaps in the iris running from the pupil margin to the iris root.

A rarer though similar deformity is a coloboma from the devlopmental fissure in the lower nasal aspect which the developing eye fails to close leaving the potential for a gap from the optic nerve head to the eyelid margin.

Adhesions between the iris and the lens frequently follow iritis. If all the way round the pupil margin, they can block the aqueous flow from the ciliary body to the anterior chamber and then the intraocular pressure will rise.

IRIS COLOURS DIFFERENT

Heterochromia

Given the complex development of the eye it is not to be wondered that occasionally the pigment distribution of the iris goes wrong. One eye green and one eye brown from birth may be odd to look at but not odd to look out from. They are of no consequence.

Pathological heterochromia

Change in the iris colour as the years go by, however, implies some pathological process. Inflammation of the ciliary body may be so low grade as to draw no attention to itself until a green iris and cataract indicate that something has been going on.

17

Double vision

At the merest suggestion of double vision, everyone is off down the brain stem trying to remember which extraocular muscle does what. Most cases of double vision do not involve the extraocular muscles at all because most images are not doubled but blurred.

Of those that are doubled, the majority occur with one eye open – *monocular diplopia*. An opacity, usually cataract, produces a ghostly second image around whatever the eye is looking at.

Of the small remainder with *genuine binocular diplopia*, most result from an imbalance of the extraocular muscles – latent squint. The eyes seek to point in a direction different from that chosen by the binocular lock. The lock may fail to stop the eyes drifting apart but it does not stop each maintaining independent vision with the inevitable result that whilst one eye looks at a chosen object, the other disturbs that choice by looking at something else.

The remainder of the small remainder are brought about by frank extraocular muscle paralysis:

- a sixth nerve palsy will limit outward movement
- a fourth nerve palsy (rare) will limit downward movement
- a third nerve palsy will limit all other movements and will cause a dropped lid *and* a dilated pupil.

All three nerves start in the brain stem and proceed to the orbit passing the cavernous sinus and the internal carotid artery on their way.

Sixth nerve (lateral rectus palsy)
Failure of one or other eye to move outwards is a not uncommon event in patients who might have some threat to their circulation, as with older diabetics, and hypertensives can suffer occlusion of the microvessels in the brain stem. The palsy usually clears up spontaneously and totally in about 6–12 weeks.

Action

Check

* the cranial nerves
* the general state of the circulation.

In young patients, poor circulation cannot be accepted as a reason for a lateral rectus palsy. The nerve, with its long pathway inside the skull, is very vulnerable to rising intracranial pressure which must be taken as likely until confirmed or disproved. Evidence might include:

* headaches that come but do not go
* swelling of the optic nerve head.

Action

Referral to a neurologist.

Fourth nerve (superior oblique) palsy
Malfunction of this muscle on its own is usually the result of trauma and the eye cannot be depressed in adduction.

Third nerve palsy
* The eyelid droops.
* The pupil is dilated.
* The eye is moved outwards and cannot move in any other direction.

The general causes are the same as with the other nerves, but sudden onset associated with pain along the distribution of the ipsilateral trigeminal nerve, must be taken as a sign of an aneurysm of the posterior communicating artery.

Action

This is a surgical emergency and calls for urgent referral to a neurosurgeon where a CT scan should confirm or refute the diagnosis of aneurysm.

Figure 17.1
Misadventure around the pituitary fossa can involve many structures. The optic nerves are vulnerable to aneurysm; the optic chiasma can be compressed by pituitary enlargement; involvement of the third, fourth, fifth and sixth nerves suggests the cavernous sinus rather than the brain stem

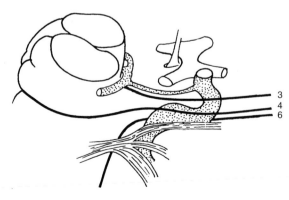

18

The normal disc and some disc anomalies

THE NORMAL DISC

Although measuring some 1.5 mm across, the normal disc appears three times larger when looked at with the direct ophthalmoscope. It is larger still in large myopic eyes and smaller in small hypermetropic eyes.

Figure 18.1
Features of a normal disc: MCC – margin, colour, cup

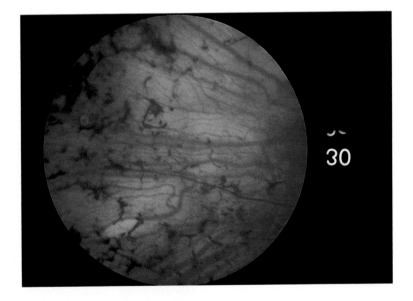

It presents three main features for which, as already explained, the letters MCC might be an aide-mémoire.

- **M** – the margin should be sharp in normal eyes but in small crowded eyes might well be blurred.
- **C** – the colour will vary according to the size of the eye – pale in the myope where the optic nerve head capillaries are more spaciously distributed, dark red in the hypermetrope for opposite reasons.

- C – the cup or cavity in the centre of the disc normally takes up about a quarter of its size. It is more precise now to talk of cup–disc ratio. With no cup present, the ratio is 0.0. If nothing but cup is present, the ratio is 0.9 or worse.

There may be a crescent on the temporal or inferior margins, particularly in short-sighted eyes where the pigment epithelium is absent. The critical thing is not to be overwhelmed by the sense of whitening all about, but to look at the colour of the disc itself.

SOME DISC ABNORMALITIES

The apparently swollen disc (pseudo papilloedema)
Small crowded eyes (long-sighted) have small crowded discs, where there is not enough room for all the normal structures to spread out.

- M – margin. It is the blurred edges that attract attention.
- C – colour. The dark redness gives the impression of swelling – an impression that must be instantly countered by the total normality of the retinal vessels and the absence of oedema and possibly haemorrhages.
- C – the cup may be absent.

Figure 18.2
Pseudo papilloedema. Like genuine papilloedema, it has no symptoms. However, normal veins, normal cranial nerves and long sight all point to a normal optic nerve head that merely gives the impression of being swollen

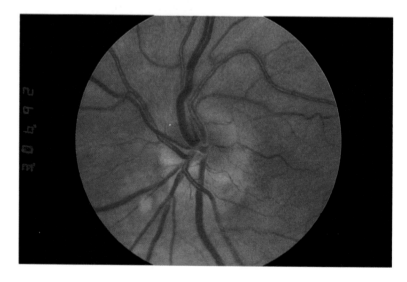

Examination

- The ophthalmic ritual. *NB: the anterior chamber in extreme long sight is very shallow and may not permit safe dilatation of the pupil.*

- The cranial nerves will reveal no abnormality.

Should doubt or anxiety remain, then the passage of the dye sodium fluorescein through the optic nerve head will reveal no abnormal leakage.

The genuinely swollen disc
- M – the margin is blurred.
- C – the colour is very red. There are also dilated veins and haemorrhages and the extension of oedema on to the adjacent retina.
- C – the cup is diminished or absent.

The retinal veins and surrounding retina join in the general engorgement and streaky retinal haemorrhage may be found as well. If papilloedema is genuine there is no visual disturbance. There may be some symptoms relating to a raised intracranial pressure.

Figure 18.3
Papilloedema. A swollen optic nerve head – characterized by blurred margins and engorged veins. If the swelling is due to papillitis, the vision will be markedly affected

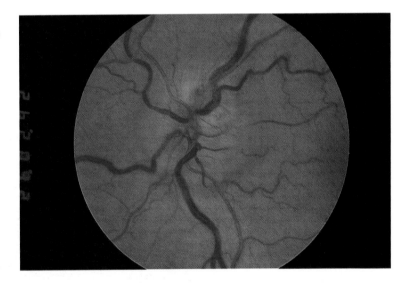

Papilloedema cannot be mistaken for venous occlusion for two reasons:

- There is no visual loss in simple papilloedema.
- The stormy sunset of the venous occlusion is unmistakable.

Papilloedema
Passive swelling of the optic nerve head is usually discovered incidentally and should have been the last thing picked up in the sequence of ophthalmic examination.

The investigation of intracranial disease has been greatly simplified by the introduction of CT scanning and taken further still by magnetic resonance imagining – MRI – which can distinguish between the different water content of different tissues, thus allowing us to demonstrate:

- oedema
- demyelination
- the results of vascular accidents.

Papillitis

To casual observation the swollen optic nerve head of papillitis differs little from that of papilloedema. The distinction lies in the impact on vision – something that would be picked up if the ophthalmic sequence were taken in order.

Unilateral papillitis is almost always due to demyelination and a large proportion of these patients will go on to develop multiple sclerosis sooner or later. *Bilateral* papillitis on the other hand is more likely to follow some viral infection.

NB: Papillitis, optic neuritis, retrobulbar neuritis are all effectively the same pathology. The difference is in their position. Retrobulbar neuritis is within the optic nerve and hence not near enough the nerve head to produce visible swelling. The impact on vision, however, is still the same.

Optic nerve head drusen

The optic nerves can swell for other reasons. Extreme reduction of intraocular pressure (hypotony) removes the mechanical support that keeps the eye in shape and a puffy disc together with retinal oedema can follow.

Drusen of the optic nerve head, hyaline material deposited in the nerve, gives a spurious impression of swelling. If nerve fibres are damaged they can produce defects not unlike those of chronic glaucoma, differing only in that they are static.

19

Squint in childhood

The eyes are moved collectively by 12 muscles, and if left without any higher control, either eye will point in any direction it chooses. The brain locks both eyes together so that both central areas join to look at one fixation point at any one time. This faculty is called binocular vision and gives us our depth perception and three-dimensional sense. Both eyes normally move with each other in near parallel when they are focused for distance. They also move against each other out of parallel when they converge to focus on something near – a reflex but recently acquired in the process of evolution and often the first to vanish when the shocks of existence become too much to bear.

Its influence can be neatly demonstrated when someone tries to catch a bouncing rugby ball with both eyes open then with one eye shut.

Eyes squint for three reasons. Because:

- there is no binocular vision
- there is binocular vision but some agency interferes with its function – such as
  (a) extraocular muscle palsy
  (b) some mechanical factor that prevents eyes from cooperating when they would like to cooperate.

EYES WITHOUT BINOCULAR VISION

Such eyes cannot be used at the same time because they point in different directions. The result is:

- the alternating use of either eye, or
- the habitual use of one eye.

The central vision of the dominant eye develops; that of the squinting eye may not. Such is the origin of amblyopia (lazy eye).

Figure 19.1
Childhood squint: the eye movements are full; there is no muscle paralysis; the angle of squint is fixed, no matter where the eyes move. The corneal reflexes are asymmetrical

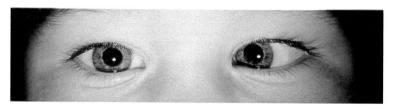

The central vision is a fragile quality before the age of 5 and many factors can arrest its development. The earlier the arrest, the deeper will be the central visual loss. Anything that blocks the direct approach of light to the central retina could bring this about.

- Opacities in the clear media, most commonly congenital cataract.
- High and sometimes different spectacle errors.
- Congenital nystagmus – denying fixation to the constantly agitated macular area.

Pseudo squint

Not all squints are in fact squints. Exaggerated skin folds from the upper lids to the nose (epicanthus), a racial characteristic in South East Asia, can give the impressions of convergence. That these folds recede spontaneously has not prevented the impatient surgeons trying to hasten their recession. Children tormented at school with the nickname of 'slit eyes' have been known to tearfully report the new one of 'scarface'.

Figure 19.2
Epicanthus. Folds of skin from the upper eyelids to the nose simulate the appearances of a converging squint. The corneal reflexes are symmetrical

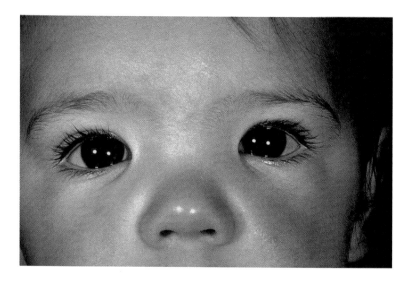

Examination

Squints that are cosmetically obvious are the best to have, because attention will be drawn to them early. The dangerous ones are the cosmetically undetectable. As unobtrusive as carcinoma of the caecum, they are discovered late.

Corneal reflexes

Each cornea behaves as a regular convex mirror throwing up a glittering reflex to the light of a pen torch. When the eyes gaze into the distance or converge equally for near, such reflexes must be symmetrical in appearance and position.

Figure 19.3
The corneal reflexes. Each cornea is a convex mirror. Reflections of a torch will occupy symmetrical positions

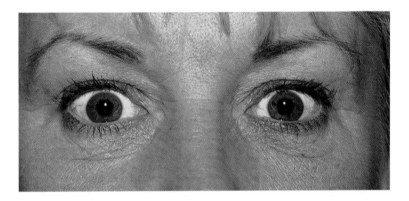

The cover test

The widespread notion that a squint must settle in one eye or the other is nonsense. Squinting eyes deviate at a fixed angle. When one eye looks straight ahead the other does not and the angle between them is the angle of the squint. If the second eye can now be persuaded to look straight ahead the first will not, and the angle between them remains the same unchanged angle of the squint.

Figure 19.4
The cover test – eyes without binocular vision: as one eye fixes the second moves inwards to converge; when the second eye moves outwards to fix, the first moves inwards to converge; the angle between them remains the same

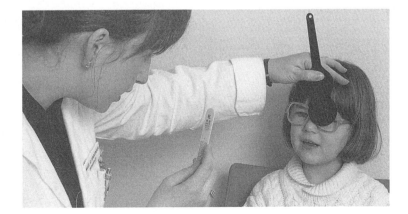

Habitual fixation with one eye does not alter this fact. It merely tells us that the macula of that side is too good ever to let go. The angle of squint still remains the fixed angle between both eyes – hence the name, concomitant squint.

The cover test is a manoeuvre to demonstrate this fixed angle. Because the test depends on fixation we must make sure the child is in fact fixing on an object of interest. By placing a hand before first one eye then the other we can demonstrate this horse rein action of both eyes as they swing at their fixed angle. The covered eye will move towards the squinting position whilst the uncovered one moves in to fix on the stick. The movements will be reversed when the hand changes eyes.

The angle remains the same; there is no muscle paralysis; the child cannot complain of double vision.

Tests for binocular vision

If binocular vision can be demonstrated then there is a very high possibility that the child does not have a squint. There are many such tests but the stereoscopic fly usually captures successfully the attention of the average 3-year-old, who will delight in trying to tear off a wing that seems to ask for such an assault.

Figure 19.5
The stereoscopic fly. Polarized glasses allow the wings to stand proud of the fly in three dimensions in the presence of normal binocular vision

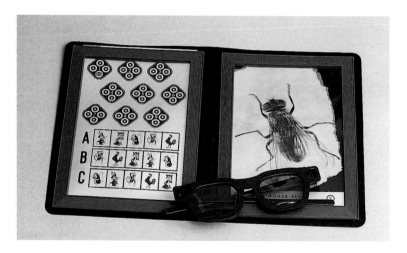

If the child has binocular vision the chances are very high that the central vision has developed and higher still that it will not undevelop.

Management
Nothing sensible can be done until:

*   appropriate glasses have been given
*   any retinal abnormality has been discovered

both with the pupils dilated.

The child is at this point handed over to the orthoptist who is well practised in wheedling information out of hostile 3-year-olds. Treatment aims to establish equal macular vision. Patching the 'good eye' during waking hours forces a functional path through to the brain. If central vision is not established by the age of 5 there is no hope for its development in the future.

Surgery
Altering the position of the eyes for cosmetic reasons is the last step in the line of treatment. In some countries where such a service is not readily available or welcome, an imposing squint is sometimes considered a token of military genius. Such dramatic qualities, often leading to tribal leadership, will not be lightly exchanged for a comely appearance.

When such prizes are not at stake, the best time for surgery is before school mates discover their talent for wounding names. Because there is no binocular lock, the eyes once straightened may continue to diverge in the same direction and eventually point outwards because the orbits point outwards anyway.

Amblyopia
The term 'lazy eye' must rival glaucoma and lasers for top place in the popular ratings of misconception. A lazy eye is physically normal, with perfect side vision but poorly developed central vision.

Anisometropic amblyopia
This is the technical term for eyes divided by large spectacle errors. They may possess the long denied capacity for binocular vision and as such want to use the eyes together.

EYES WITH BINOCULAR VISION

Extraocular muscle palsy
Whatever the underlying cause, a paralysed muscle in a conscious patient who has developed binocular vision must produce double vision.

NB: Patients frequently complain of double vision when they really mean blurred vision.

The younger age groups
Muscle palsy must always be taken seriously, whether of sudden or languid onset.

Latent squint

In nobody are the eyes absolutely straight. However, the slight hidden deviations are always overcome by a powerful binocular lock. Such deviations become apparent when the eyes prefer to separate from each other more than the binocular lock can tolerate. Symptoms of fleeting double vision and difficulty in depth perception depend on how quickly such people can pull their eyes together again. If another stress is added then the lock may just break apart. A classic example of this came to light during the Second World War when certain pilots found it impossible to judge the position of the runway – an understandable lapse of judgement given the relief that they had survived once more and might not survive next time.

Examination

The cover/uncover test
This test of binocular function tells us two things:

- How far the eye has to travel to get back into position.
- How well and how quickly it travels.

Figure 19.6
The cover/uncover test for latent squint. When covered, the left eye diverges. When the cover is removed the binocular lock pulls it back into position again

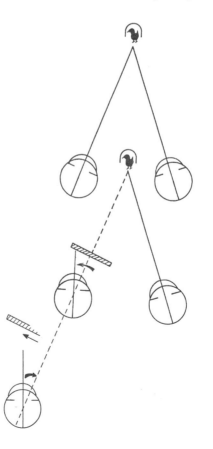

With the binocular lock broken by an occluding hand, the covered eye drifts into its natural aberrant position. With the hand removed and the lock restored, the eye returns to where it should be.

Symptoms arise when the distance to travel is long and the time to travel is slow.

Action

- Orthoptic exercises make the patient feel better while leaving the deviation very much as it was.
- Prismatic glasses move the viewed image to the deviating eye which in time deviates even more.
- Surgery may well be needed to reduce a gross separation.

Convergence weakness

The convergence reflex, a most recent acquisition, is usually the first to disintegrate under stress. Stress varies according to one's interests, but the thought of studying on a hot summer evening or imminent exposure at an examination may induce young people from time to time to develop double vision for near objects.

There is no extraocular muscle palsy, the eyes just cannot converge to read. Today, simple orthoptic exercises help bring the convergence a point nearer to the nose. In the days before package holidays, textbooks on refraction would often recommend a winter by the Jungfrau. It is conceivable that after the inevitable broken leg, convergence might have recovered swiftly, with reading the only relief from boredom.

20

Trauma

Injuries to the face frequently look worse than they are and careless description often talks of the 'eye' when just about everything else but the eye is affected.

The first concern is whether or not the eye itself is involved. The second concern may not appear significant until months or years later when:

- The intraocular pressure creeps up unnoticed.
- The retina, torn at its anterior edge, begins slowly to detach.

The essential question to ask is: **'Was anything travelling fast enough to penetrate the eye?'**

Even with a slit lamp, this may often still be an example of a condition best diagnosed from the history. All manner of substances may enter the eye. Wood splinters, as discovered during the days of the wooden wall battleships, are particularly infective. Metal fragments oxidize and deposits of metallic salts through the globe, changing the colour of the iris, eventually destroy the ciliary body.

Out of horror can sometimes come benefit. The whole magic tale of lens implantation began with the observation in injured pilots that intraocular fragments of aircraft perspex remained inert and did not chemically destroy the eye.

THE EYELIDS

Laceration of a lid margin is particularly dangerous.

Figure 20.1
Repair of a lid margin laceration
must take precedence over
everything except actual laceration
of the globe itself

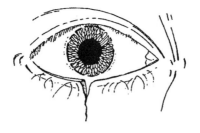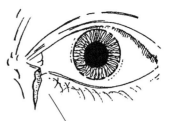

Lower canaliculus threatened

Action

Short term: Since the instant problem is exposure and irritation, closure of the lid with adhesive tape over lubricating ointment will protect the globe.
Long term: Surgical reconstruction demands precise apposition of the torn lid margins.

THE EYEBALL

Damage may be:

- laceration
- contusion
- chemical.

• LACERATION

A rent in the outer wall of the eye is usually easily recognized. It is equally easy for an infection to enter and, with careless handling, easy for the contents of the eye to be expelled.

Action

Short term:

- avoid pressure on the globe
- topical antibiotics
- protective shield
- urgent referral.

Figure 20.2
Prolapsed iris

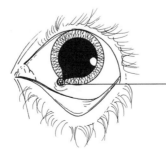

Limbal rupture and
iris prolapse

Figure 20.3
The iris: whatever colour it seems to
have inside the eye is always black
when prolapsed

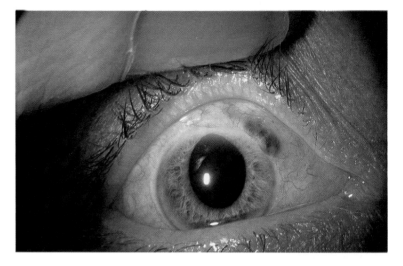

- CONTUSION
Trauma anywhere causes:

- bleeding and instant damage to vital structures
- long term inflammatory damage to everything.

Hyphaema
Blood in the anterior chamber is recognized by a fluid level
that settles out rather like cells in an ESR tube. If the
hyphaema is total, the inevitable raised pressure squeezes
blood into the corneal stroma, where it remains as a visually
disabling yellow stain.

Figure 20.4
Hyphaema: blood in the anterior
chamber, usually the result of
trauma. The eye is irritable and a
further haemorrhage can: fill the
anterior chamber; block the drain
and raise the pressure; block the
drainage angle; raise the pressure;
stain the cornea

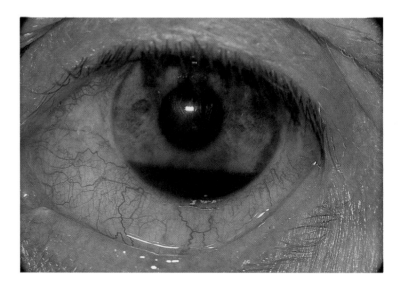

Action

Short term:

- bed rest can prevent secondary haemorrhage, which would appear to lead to this catastrophe
- topical corticosteroids suppress the inflammation
- raised pressure and increase in hyphaema demand that the blood be evacuated – urgently.

Long term: late sequelae of blunt trauma can take many years to develop:

Figure 20.5
A blow severe enough to have caused a hyphaema can also: dislocate the lens; tear the retina; reduce drainage with late rise in intraocular pressure

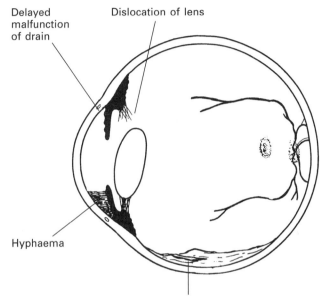

Delayed malfunction of drain

Dislocation of lens

Hyphaema

Tear in peripheral retina

- The intraocular pressure can rise.
- Secondary fibrosis blocks the drainage angle.
- The retina can detach from peripheral tears sustained during the original blow, so long after the event, that the connection may not be suspected.
- A lens may survive dislocation but not always cataract formation.

A good rule is that a blow sufficient to cause hyphaema can:

- rupture the globe
- dislocate the lens
- tear the peripheral retina
- raise the intraocular pressure.

The first step to diagnosis and management is to consider these things possible.

• CHEMICAL

The range is bewildering, but strong acids and alkalis are familiar substitutes for the gun. Both chemicals cause lethal damage. They:

• destroy the conjunctiva
• deform the lids, causing them to adhere to the eye
• turn in the lashes
• opacify the cornea
• scarify the drainage angle.

Action

The only recourse is to flood the eye with water as soon as possible.

THE ORBIT

A blow-out fracture of the orbital floor or wall is a familiar weekend injury, often occurring when the victim's perception is not at its highest. With the orbital contents trapped (usually) in the maxillary sinus, the eye will move neither upwards nor downwards and if the condition is neglected will never do so freely in the future.

Figure 20.6
Blow-out fracture. If the orbit and eye are too swollen to allow detailed examination, loss of sensation over the cheek would suggest trapping of the maxillary nerve in the orbital floor. A blow sufficient to rupture the orbital floor can do the same to the eye

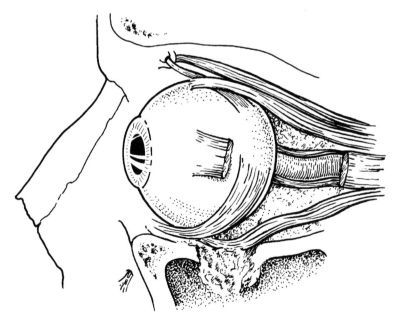

Action

The ophthalmic ritual clearly has to be curtailed, but if the right and left cornea, pupils and anterior chambers resemble each other, then the chances are that the eye has not been ruptured. Radiographic examination will confirm or refute any clinical impression.

Various manoeuvres are now available to release the entrapped muscle.

SYMPATHETIC OPHTHALMITIS

Penetrating injury, particularly one involving the lens, iris and ciliary body, can stimulate the production of circulating antibodies to normal eye tissue. They fail to recognize the eye as 'self' and, brought into being by one eye, end up destroying both. The result is a smouldering pan-uveitis.

Because the condition is happily rare, it is not easy to establish guidelines in practice. Renewed pain in a red, watering eye would be accepted as a symptom that should not be ignored.

Should the exciting eye be damaged with no hope of useful vision, then enucleation may save the fellow from any involvement. The dilemma starts when the inflamed eye has useful vision as well as all the signs of sympathetic ophthalmitis. At this point we dare not remove it because it may end up the better eye.

21

The vascular retinopathies

Malfunction of the retinal blood vessels provides yet another demonstration that the eye is a one-response organ. Blood vessels, whose normal function can appear so remarkable until it fails, can be incompetent in many ways and under many influences:

- Idiopathic – hypertension
- Inflammatory – the collagen disorders
- Metabolic – diabetes
- Diminished blood flow – carotid occlusive disease.

Figure 21.1
How vascular disorders can affect the eye

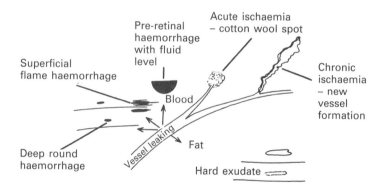

Figure 21.2
Retinal haemorrhages. These are diagnostic of nothing other than bleeding from a variety of causes

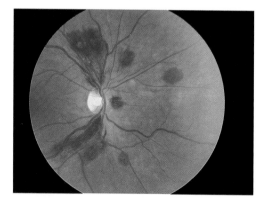

There are others, which merely serve to confirm the fact that the common end point of them all is capillary inefficiency which will result in:

- leakage – of
  (a) plasma – hard exudates
  (b) blood – haemorrhages – round in the deep layers, flame-shaped in the superficial layers, formless in the vitreal cavity
- diminished blood flow (ischaemia).

The retina has only one response to ischaemia, no matter what its cause. It produces new blood vessels, presumably in search of more oxygen but unfortunately in receipt of blood.

DIMINISHED BLOOD FLOW

Optic nerve head and peripheral retina

Blood vessels on the optic nerve head, because of their fragility, are useless providers of oxygen but are very effective at rupturing into the vitreal cavity. The very act of bleeding, seems to stimulate some proliferative factor that encourages the growth of fibrous membranes which adhere to the surface of the retina. Such membranes then shrink and pucker, pulling the retina into the vitreal cavity where, if left, it will, like all other starving brain tissue, become functionless.

Figure 21.3
New vessels on the optic nerve head – a non-specific response to ischaemia

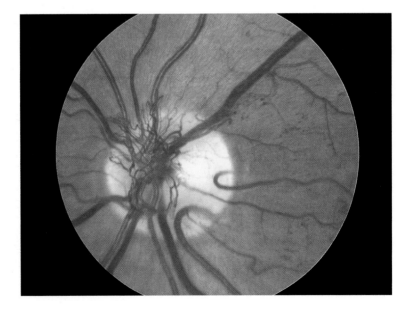

Iris

In extreme forms of ischaemia, these vessels develop over the iris, doing nothing for the overall oxygenation of the eye, but completely blocking the flow of aqueous through the trabecular meshwork (rubeosis). Because the pressure rises suddenly, the eye becomes painful and red and frequently defies all attempts to bring the pressure down again.

It is traditional to describe the various retinopathies under the different headings and there indeed are *one or two differences*, but the underlying pattern is common to all because the retina, like every other part of the eye, has one response.

22

Hypertension

The response of the eye to a rising blood pressure, like so much else in ophthalmology, can be made incomprehensible over several chapters – or it can be reduced to its three essential elements:

- The starting state of the vessels.
- The rate of hypertensive change.
- The extent of hypertensive change.

- THE STATE OF THE BLOOD VESSELS

In the childhood eye the retinal venules and arterioles are of equal width and both are well endowed with elastic tissue, and the arterioles also with muscle. They glisten regularly in the light of an ophthalmoscope. As the circulation pulses normally over the years, the elastic and muscles are replaced by fibrous tissue which dulls the glistening reflex. The calibre of the arterioles becomes slightly reduced and the shifting highlights of the young retina give way to a dry coarse mottling. When the age of decline arrives, these fibrotic changes may, without offence, be given the name of involutionary sclerosis.

Figure 22.1
In a child the arterioles and venules are of equal width and the background retina glistens. In an adult, the arterioles are more narrow. The background loses the sparkle of youth

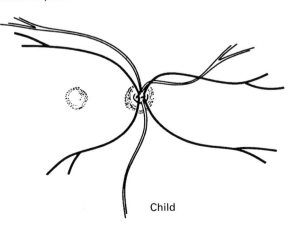

Child

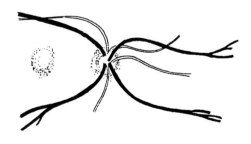

Adult

The fundamental point is that when the blood pressure rises, the retinal vessels of the young eye, full of elastic tissue and muscle, will behave very differently from the rigid fibrotic vessels of an older eye.

- ## RATE AND EXTENT OF CHANGE

Gradual rise

In the **ageing eye**, all the changes of age become exaggerated. Remaining arteriolar muscle goes into spasm. The fibrotic elements remain as they were or even dilate somewhat, giving rise to 'arteriolar calibre variation'.

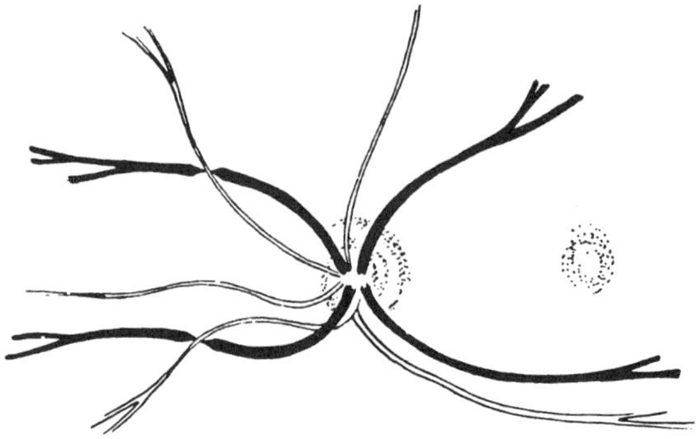

Figure 22.2
Nipping of the arteriovenous (AV) crossing is the first evidence in the eye of a raised blood pressure. The first evidence, however, must surely be picked up in the arm

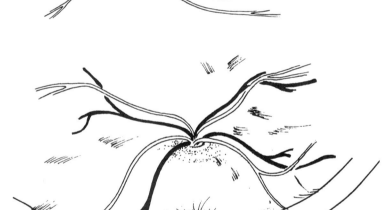

Figure 22.3
Arteriovenous (AV) crossing changes, scattered flame haemorrhages and exudates at the macula in a star pattern, are findings classically associated with hypertension

All these changes can be picked up with the direct ophthalmoscope. Should the ophthalmoscope begin to fail, other features can be picked up as well. The celebrated shift in the arteriolar reflex from silver to copper is not a clinical sign, but rather one of battery failure. None the less, it keeps turning up in textbook after textbook, like a rich aunt whom no one dare exclude from the wedding list.

The arterioles begin to give the impression of nipping the veins where they cross and these arteriovenous (AV) changes are recognized as the first sign that hypertension has begun to turn an appearance of age into a disease.

In the youthful eye young vessels respond to a leisurely rise in blood pressure with involutionary change, which although physiological at 60, is pathological at 20.

In both age groups, the capillaries eventually begin to leak lipids and formed blood into the surrounding tissue.

Rapid rise

In the **ageing eye**, all the changes of age just described form with greater speed and indeed occasionally with savage rapidity. Involutionary fibrosis actually protects the vessels against the effect of severe pressure elevation.

Without protective fibrosis, in the **youthful eye** the arterioles go into spasm. The retina becomes swollen and the blood pressure reading may go off the scale.

Fluffy white patches (cotton wool spots), brought about by retinal ischaemia, appear at random. The haemorrhages of simple hypertension become more florid and may burst into the vitreous. The optic nerve head swells – papilloedema (malignant hypertension).

Grading

Perfectly sensible attempts to describe hypertensive change in shorthand come to grief because we can never be sure that other people are using the same system. We end by adding a number to what is already perfectly simple to describe – an additional detail to be forgotten before it is understood.

• COMPLICATIONS

Occlusion of the central retinal artery

Interruption to the arterial flow leads to total infarction of the retina which, normally transparent, becomes white and opaque except at the macula, where it is thin enough to allow the choroid to be seen (cherry red spot).

In time the retina becomes transparent again. The red reflex returns but, alas, the vision does not. Neither does the red glow return to the optic nerve head, which whitens into optic atrophy.

Because the retina is anoxic rather than hypoxic, and there is no half-dead tissue desperate for oxygen, new blood vessels do not appear.

Occlusion of the central retinal vein

Flame haemorrhages stretch across the retina like blood red clouds at dusk, whilst the swollen veins coil back through the stormy sunset to an equally swollen optic nerve head. If the retina is hypoxic (particularly so when the central vision is damaged) the eye will make its habitual single response, with fragile blood vessels sprouting over the retina and over the iris root where they bring the aqueous flow to a halt, usually irreversibly.

Figure 22.4
Central retinal vein occlusion. The stormy sunset of central vision, more likely in connection with: chronic simple glaucoma; hypertension; diabetes. Hyperviscosity must be excluded as a matter of course

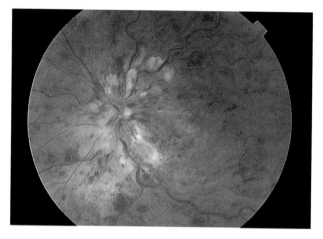

Although we can predict and try to explain this varying florid painful response to hypoxia, we do not actually know *why it happens*. At least we know *when*, and call it the hundred day glaucoma. The name is apt and recalls the time that passed between Napoleon's flight from Elba and the final blood bath at Waterloo. As for the swollen veins, they conjure forth images of elderly statesmen at the Congress of Vienna, fully occupied, doing not very much, suddenly apoplectic at the news that the Emperor of the French was once more in Paris.

Central retinal vein occlusion is a frequent associate of chronic simple glaucoma and indeed may be a presenting sign.

Vitreal haemorrhage

Fragile capillaries rupturing into the vitreal cavity sometimes clear briefly to reveal no actual source of bleeding, before a fresh flood of haemorrhage obscures the fundus once again.

There are other causes of bleeding into the vitreous:

* diabetes
* retinal break (and detachment).

Hypertension is the 'chronic glaucoma' of medicine. Patients almost never know they have it until some vital function is lost.

23

Diabetic retinopathy

In the United Kingdom there are about 1 million diabetics: 20% are insulin dependent, 80% are maturity onset, and for every person known to have the disease, there is another one undiagnosed. Although ocular complications become more common over time, other factors hasten their development.

Figure 23.1
Retinopathy that happens to be due to diabetes. The prelude to catastrophe for eyes that may well, at this stage, be without symptoms

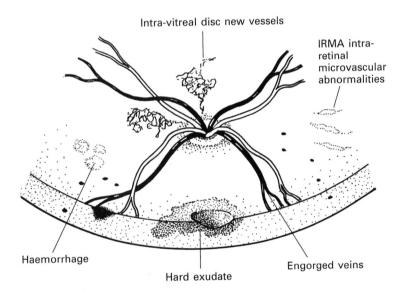

Intra-vitreal disc new vessels

IRMA intra-retinal microvascular abnormalities

Haemorrhage

Hard exudate

Engorged veins

High levels of glycosylated haemoglobin (A1), particularly in insulin dependents, indicating casual control of blood sugar, accelerates the onset of microvascular complications. Non-insulin dependents are especially at risk because they may not know for several years that they have diabetes. The clinical response of both groups is the same.

Microaneurysms
These outpouchings from the weakened walls of small vessels are specific to diabetes.

Thereafter, the sequence of:

- retinal haemorrhages
- retinal exudates

develops as with any vascular retinopathy.

Ischaemia (hypoxia)

Venous changes
Distortion and dilatation of the retinal veins, which in themselves are not very dramatic, are the first clear signs that the retinal blood supply is not coping with the demands.

Cotton wool spots
Formerly known as soft exudates, these spots are another unmistakable sign of even more severe retinal ischaemia. They might be regarded as retinal infarcts but they are actual accumulations of axonal transport material, accumulating because flow in the nerves has come to a halt.

Figure 23.2
The so-called background diabetic retinopathy. Poor circulation indicated by: dilated veins; leakage of blood (haemorrhages); leakage of fat (exudates)

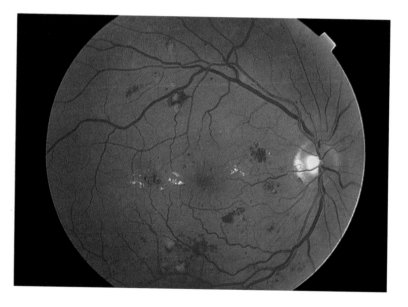

Intra-retinal microvascular abnormality (IRMA)
Such dilated capillaries can be picked up with the direct ophthalmoscope, the green filter of which eliminates the red of the choroid and makes it possible to outline these elongated dilatations in black against a pale green background. Together with venous changes, extensive intra-retinal haemorrhage and cotton wool spots, they indicate that the retina has now entered the pre-proliferative phase.

Proliferation

Severe hypoxia stimulates the retina to seek other sources of oxygen. The creation of new vessels has already been described, together with the process by which haemorrhage into the vitreal gel stimulates fibrosis, which in turn ends as a fine membrane, adherent to the retinal surface, wrinkling, puckering, shrinking and pulling the retina into all manner of patterns, and indeed pulling it off altogether.

Figure 23.3
The start of proliferation. The appearances of general retinal health are proved delusive by: (i) new vessels on the optic nerve head; (ii) fibrosis in the vitreous with proliferal new retinal vessel formation. Untreated, this is the high road to disaster

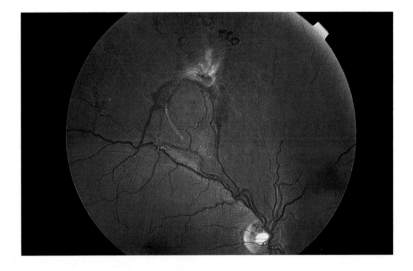

Any diabetic retinal change, no matter how bland it looks at one visit, is capable of threatening sight before the next.

Intravenous fluorescein angiography

Sodium fluorescein, the same dye used to pick up deficiencies in the corneal epithelium, can be photographed as it passes through the eye after injection into an arm vein.

Irradiation with blue light induces fluorescence of the dye which, collecting where it should not and lingering when it ought not, can reveal:

- gaps and cracks in the ocular layers – together with
- leaks stasis and closure in the choroidal and retinal circulations.

MANAGEMENT

- Good diabetic control.
- Regular examination of the fundus through the dilated pupil (every 6 months).
- Light coagulation (laser).
- Vitrectomy.

Laser

The laser is a destructive instrument, used in the hope that the preservation of functioning retinal tissue will more than compensate for its conversion of dying retinal tissue to dead. The coagulating light is picked up by the retinal pigment epithelium and converted to heat, which coagulates and destroys anything in contact with it. Clearly it cannot be used in the presence of a retinal detachment, although the tabloid press would have us believe it can.

Figure 23.4
Treated diabetic retinopathy – widespread chorioretinal scars brought about by laser photocoagulation. The characteristic feature is their distribution. Each on its own, however, has all the other features that make all chorioretinal scars look the same – white sclera shining through patches of atrophic choroid and scattered pigment

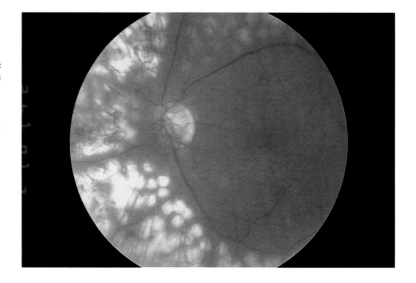

Macular dysfunction

The light can be delivered either:

*   in a grid pattern to reduce widespread oedema – or
*   in a focal pattern, closing off discrete sources of leakage or haemorrhage.

Proliferation

Background features such as microaneurysms and round haemorrhages may go on for many years. The warning bells of pre-proliferation should begin to sound where cotton wool spots and IRMA begin to dominate in a now wet-looking retina between increasingly dilated veins.

Something more radical with the same laser is now required. It was observed that diabetics with widespread spontaneous scarring from whatever cause tended not to develop proliferative eye disease. It was further observed that inducing such scars with some form of coagulation had the same effect. It is now customary to induce a scatter of laser burns over the retina. In theory, the substitution of anoxic for hypoxic retina balances the level of oxygen required to the level of oxygen available, thus reducing the stimulus to the formation of new blood vessels.

Vitrectomy
Many eyes that in the past used to end up blind and painful can now be salvaged by entering the posterior cavity of the eye with a vitreal suction cutter, intravitreal forceps and scissors, endodiathermy and endolaser and a whole series of foreign agents:

- air or expanding gas
- heavy liquids
- silicone oil.

Such intervention, becoming with increasing usage standard rather than heroic, has brought hope and vision where before there was only blindness. Doubtless in time some further biochemical advance with a metabolic magic bullet, will make vitrectomy as dated as pituitary ablation.

24

Other vascular anomalies

AIDS

Like syphilis, AIDS is the great simulator, attacking aggressively without apparent restraint any bodily system, and it is not surprising that asymptomatic transient disturbances of the retinal microvascular circulation commonly occur. The retinal changes are not pathognomonic of AIDS; they are merely pathognomonic of retinal changes that occur in response to circulatory disturbance whatever the cause.

This is in line with the eye's standard behaviour of having a limited response, indeed almost the same response, to a multiplicity of different agencies. The changes are faintly reminiscent of those found in diabetic retinopathy, and in a sense follow the same pattern, but clearly the exciting reason is different.

Retinopathy of prematurity

The identical clinical picture under the name of retrolental fibroplasia has been identified as a response to excessive exposure to oxygen after birth. It was quietly drifting into the chapters of history when the neonatologists resurrected it under its present title. In normal circumstances, blood vessels grow in an ordered pattern in the retina and from the retina to the ora serrata. When this order is disturbed then the threat of retinal disorganization can be added to all the other possible organ defects facing premature children.

Time-consuming recurrent examination of these children in the exhausting temperature of the neonatal intensive care unit has to be carried out during the first 12 weeks of life.

Cryotherapy or laser photocoagulation, both under general anaesthesia, may save a certain proportion of these eyes.

This condition neatly encapsulates the medical dilemma that the elimination of one major scourge can give rise to more than one in its wake.

25

Retinoblastoma

This growth is fortunately as rare as it is malignant, occurring once in more than 20,000 live births. Its favourite site of origin is the posterior retina. It rapidly fills the vitreous with tumour seedlings, which whiten the normal black pupil. It is this feature, and perhaps the occasional squint, rather than visual loss which captures parental notice.

Most cases occur before the age of 3 and there is a one in three chance that both eyes may be affected.

Action

Enucleation is obligatory for large tumours but smaller ones may be attacked by a combination of radiotherapy and chemotherapy – very successfully.

In known families, the heredity appears to be an autosomal dominant with 80% penetrance. In practical terms this means that half the children will carry the trait and of this half, four out of five will suffer the disease.

Where there is no family history it would appear that most cases are sporadic and the offspring of these children who survive successful surgery do not seem to demonstrate any dominant hereditary pattern.

26

Management of refractive errors

There is no greater victim of alternative remedies than an eye that might see better with glasses. The simplest way to deal with such an optically deficient eye is to pretend that the second rate vision is normal. There has been no shortage of mountebanks who preach that to wear glasses is to depend on them. They offer ethereal lens-free vision to myopes, presbyopes, hypermetropes and astigmatics who, completely fog bound, are prepared to blunder their way to the natural life.

These zealots forget that their own shoes, clothes, dental fillings and hearing aids should also be denounced as an outrage against nature. Yet nobody would deny that we walk better with shoes, appear better with clothes, bite better with intact teeth and hear better with hearing aids. If glasses are needed, we will see better with them. The dependence is not on glasses but on the pleasure of seeing.

Yet books are still written to persuade the credulous that an act of will may transform a weakness that they were born with into a strength that they would like. Other healers accept the optical defect but recommend nature cures. The technique of palming might come into this category, and its underlying principles are wonderously simple. If we cannot see properly, we press the palms of our hands firmly on to the eyes, uncovering them to see better and then covering them again if we cannot. The process is repeated indefinitely. The beauty of the system is how well the eyes can see when the hands are removed – provided there is nothing wrong with them. And in extreme errors of refraction, the technique is never put to the test because the hands are not off the eyes for long enough to reveal a failed miracle.

Poor vision has nothing to recommend it at any time, but particularly when inflicted on the gullible, terrorized out of a pair of glasses in exchange for the bogus alternative of visual paradise.

But visions of paradise were not in the minds of the ecclesiastical authorities when they opposed the concept of correcting lenses. The man credited with their introduction was a Franciscan monk called Roger Bacon, although his primary interest was to speculate on the qualities of light, an activity that brought with it accusations of witchcraft. Like so many of those contributions that have benefited the world, his work was regarded as heresy by the hierarchy of the Church, whose main interest was the preservation of the status quo. They took a rather dim view of his experiments, and indeed many of them did so literally, because they might well have used his discoveries to their advantage.

Although a Jesuit priest rather later has been given the credit for discovering the pinhole, it is probable that Roger Bacon got there first. Doubtless he thought the better of publishing the products of his labours to an audience whose disapproval might have resulted in more than his career going up in a puff of smoke.

The first correcting lenses to be mass produced in the fourteenth century were convex, correcting the long-sighted eye for distance and the presbyope for near. In due course concave lenses for myopia became equally available, though it is probable that myopes, seeing clearly only for near, had a shorter lifespan because longevity would depend on seeing in the distance dangers that might shorten life when unsuspected until close at hand.

The short-sighted eye can never see in the distance at any time with or without effort, and of all the many world famous myopes none was more famous or more myopic than Sir George Brown, of the Crimean High Command. Even Lord Raglan, the Commander in Chief, whose only attempt to read a novel ended after thirty pages, considered him to be lacking in imagination. Yet he did have the insight to recognize that his failure to see either army could have no influence on the course of the campaign. As it turned out, it had more than he could ever have imagined. His chosen line of advance took his brigade at right-angles to that chosen by Lord Raglan. The Russians on the heights of the Alma, gazing in wonder at this rabble, advancing in the shape of a cross, took it for a new military formation divinely inspired and fled. Had Sir George the distance vision to see his triumph, without doubt he would have created a disaster instead.

As well as optical devices for looking through, there are also those for looking well with, whilst looking through. The lorgnette favoured by Beau Brummell and the Scarlet Pimpernel belong to this category. It is inconceivable that anyone so perfect as either would actually have required any sort of correction, either for long sight or short sight, and certainly they would not have admitted it openly. In these circumstances, the lorgnette became simply a partition to separate the disdaining from the disdained.

The single lens on a handle – the quizzing glass – served very much the same purpose, doubtless allowing the uncorrected eye to do the actual seeing. With the handle discarded, the quizzing glass becomes a monocle held in place by the action of the facial muscles. Although popularly associated with caricatures of Prussian officers, it was in fact an essential adjunct to female fashion around 1816. When the havoc wrought in the skin around the orbits became too much like crows' feet to be ignored the fashion was quietly dropped, leaving the glass screwed firmly into the eyelids of the stage Prussian, where it has stayed ever since.

A refugee doctor from central Europe after the Second World War, answering a question in the Diploma of Ophthalmology, was clearly of this belief when he said: 'I do not know what the optical principles of the monocle are, but I do know it was adopted by the Gestapo to strike fear into the hearts of subject people.'

When spectacles fail, the surgeon's approach to most things is generally to produce a knife, and at the extremes of visual inadequacy several surgical approaches have been devised. Before that, however, we have to consider contact lenses.

Contact lenses

Contact lenses are foreign bodies applied to the cornea in the hope that visual betterment or emotional relief from discarding spectacles will compensate for the insult to the eye of their application. Made from a variety of synthetic transparent materials of differing physical attributes, they are accepted by the eye only in the presence of a normal fluid exchange across the corneal surface and an adequate supply of tears.

These conditions are not always met. Fluid balance throughout the body fluctuates as the normal hormonal cycles fluctuate, and when these cycles are further unbalanced by the contraceptive pill, pregnancy or impending abortion, intolerance of contact lenses may be the first indication. Should the tear secretion decline below a certain critical level, then this intolerance becomes permanent.

Even healthy eyes have their problems. Coarsely fitted lenses depriving the anterior corneal surface of oxygen will cause a hazy oedema of the epithelium. Over-wearing of well-fitted lenses will produce the same result, and if carried to foolish lengths may induce the growth of superficial new vessels around the corneoscleral limbus – presumably to make up the oxygen normally supplied by the tears.

With this baleful array of hazards it is a wonder that people wear contact lenses at all. They do so for a variety of reasons. Vanity and cosmetic satisfaction can lead to a tolerance of the most appalling discomforts, and most contact lenses are worn for these reasons. A quality contact lens fitted by an expert does not produce appalling discomfort and there can be no doubt that eyes with extreme refractive errors see more effectively with such lenses than they do with standard glasses.

The visual field enlarges when unhampered by thick spectacle frames, and the distorting periphery of a thick lens is not used when a lens of equivalent strength is placed upon the eye. Central vision also sharpens, because contact with the eye is a much more natural arrangement than glasses in a frame. The pity is that it is not a more natural corneal arrangement.

Such lenses have their uses for medical reasons. Unilateral aphakics who have normal vision in the other eye may regain binocular function when a contact lens comes near to restoring the optical balance of the eye to what it was before the cataract was removed.

The increasing use of intraocular lens implants has at the moment almost eliminated the optical difficulties of unilateral aphakia.

An abnormal curvature of the cornea (keratoconus) not only induces myopia, but also thin opaque corneal stroma at the summit of the cone. A judiciously designed lens may not only prevent this disaster, but may improve the vision as well and delay the need for corneal grafting. Although it may seem paradoxical, there is some evidence that contact lenses, far from delaying the progression of keratoconus, can actually hasten it.

When corneal ulcers refuse to heal, stitching the eyelids together (tarsorrhaphy) is not always acceptable, especially in an only eye. A contact lens can be applied as a bandage to allow the corneal epithelium to regenerate without external disturbance. The lids stay open, the patient may continue to see, and the sceptical will also see that covering the cornea is not just a device to conceal therapeutic defeat.

Contact lens wearers complain from time to time of irritable eyes. This is not surprising as the potential cause has been applied by themselves. Corneal abrasions, erosions, infections and frank assault from trying to remove a contact lens that may not be in position are all ways in which this may happen. More common is a grumbling conjunctivitis caused by simple intolerance to the lens material, or allergy to the endless variety of solutions available for them to steep in.

Most symptoms will clear away when the lens is taken out. Most symptoms will stay away if the lens is kept out, at least until the signs and any doubts over its suitability have cleared away as well.

Surgical correction

Given the prevalence of extreme myopia in Japan, even amongst air crew, it was necessary during the Second World War to find an optical correction that did not continue in one direction whilst the plane had turned sharply in another. The first surgical attempt to alter the corneal curvature was made by a Japanese eye surgeon – Sato – to overcome not only the lack of distance vision in the Japanese pilots but also a lack of the actual pilots themselves. His incisions were placed on the deep surface of the cornea. It can only be guessed what long term effect this might have had on the endothelium because the *kamikaze* principle did not make for long careers in the air, but at least, it spared the pilots the ghastly realization that if they had not given up their lives for their Emperor, they would certainly have given up their eyes.

During the 1970s, Fyodorov, in what was then the Soviet Union, modified this approach to changing the corneal shape by making his attack on the outer surface of the cornea. A computer, fed with appropriate information, instructs the surgeon who then makes a series of radial incisions around an axial circle as far as the deep corneal layer, and sometimes, alas, beyond.

Figure 26.1
The correction for short sight. The most common is not to correct it at all, settling for an impressionist's view of the distance, improved to a degree by narrowing of the eyelid aperture

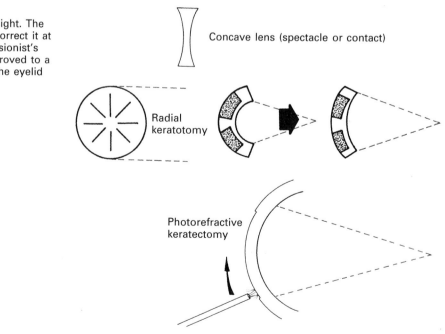

As can be guessed, the stratagem is not without its drawbacks. Unpleasant reflections can bounce into the eye from the surgical interfaces, which act as mirrors. The resultant photophobia might then induce a twinge of regret for the comfortable old glasses, or even the contact lenses. If only it were as effective in severe myopia, it would be accepted without reservation. On the present evidence, it can only be a matter of time before radial keratotomy becomes part of history, like the Mensheviks, an essential catalyst to the start of a revolution, anticipating a new world in which they would play no part.

Photorefractive keratectomy (PRK)
The Excimer laser is the next step in what doubtless will be a sequence of increasing sophistication. The aim is still to reduce the corneal curvature but without the brutal penetration of its stroma required by radial keratotomy.

With great precision and relative freedom from discomfort, the cornea can be fashioned, within reason, to eliminate spherical or astigmatic refractive errors up to a level of 6 dioptres.

Laser in situ kerato-mileusis (Lasik)
There is a limit beyond which simple sculpting may well produce a more desirable refractive error but unfortunately will produce a hazy cornea as well. In these cases, the appropriate refraction is sculpted beneath a mobilized Bowman's membrane and epithelium.

Both PRK and Lasik are usually carried out on patients who would like to improve on a vision that may in fact be already at a high level. As can be guessed, their sense of success and response to the result may be more critical than that of patients whose only desire is to see again.

Phototherapeutic keratectomy (PTK)
The Excimer laser also has a place in the removal of corneal opacities with a precision that cannot be matched by any scalpel.

Intraocular manipulations
In a very high degree of myopia, surgeons have been moved to counter the strong focusing power of the natural lens with a concave implant into the anterior chamber. An equal surgical interest has been directed at the natural lens itself. Removal of a clear lens, not yet a cataract, reduces the optical myopia enormously but of course does nothing to alter the degenerative areas of myopia that may exist in such eyes.

Both approaches are invasive, with all the possible complications of surgical invasion of the eye possibly made more distressing by the flimsy surgical indications that led to them.

27

Visual standards

Blind registration
Although the definition by statute splits into three sections, consideration of all three does not lead to improved understanding. In essence, qualification depends on the balance between:

- the level of central vision, and
- constriction of the visual field.

  Patients are eligible when:

- the central vision is less than 3/60 irrespective of the state of the visual field, or
- the central vision is less than 6/60 with a constricted visual field.

Partial sight
No absolute level of vision has been defined by statute, but by common usage it is accepted that:

- the central vision should be 6/24 or less, associated with
- some constriction of the visual field.

  Being monocular does not qualify for the partial sight register. The monocular subject could well drive a Ferrari for pleasure (private vehicle licence) but not as a taxi (public vehicle licence).

Standards for driving
Drivers may hold a private licence provided:

- they can make out on a motor vehicle registration plate, letters of 79.4 mm in height at a distance of 20.5 m. (In practical terms this means a central vision of between 6/12 and 6/9.)

- Their visual field spreads as a rectangle
  (a) at least 120 degrees in the horizontal meridian and
  (b) 20 degrees above and 20 degrees below fixation in the vertical meridian
  (c) without any defect in the inner quality (scotoma) closer than 10 degrees to fixation.

Public service vehicles (and heavy goods vehicle) licence
The essential difference here is that such drivers are required to have two eyes unless they held a heavy goods vehicle licence before such a requirement was obligatory. Such drivers should in addition:

- possess an ordinary driving licence
- achieve 3/60 unaided with each eye separately and 6/9 corrected with the poorer eye being not less than 6/12
- have no insuperable double vision
- have no field defect.

There are some variations between the requirements for a heavy goods vehicle and a metropolitan taxi cab but they are so subtle that any attempt to find a distinction may result in our being baffled by both.

28

Miscellany of words, drugs and rarities

accommodation mechanism by which the eye changes focus, essentially from distance to near. Contraction of the ciliary muscle alters the shape of the lens. The act of accommodation produces constriction of the pupil.

acyclovir has eclipsed idoxuridine in the treatment of herpes simplex infections and has transformed the management of herpes zoster. A variant, gancyclovir, may not have transformed the management of AIDS but does have a useful place.

adrenalin *see* mydriatics

agnosia failure to recognize familiar objects despite intact vision.

albinism the retinal pigment layer plays a vital function in the metabolism of visual pigments as well as absorbing excess light. It is recognized by the classic bleach-white skin and hair of the albino, and the red reflex which can be seen not only through the pupil but through the atrophic iris as well.

Figure 28.1
Albinism. Fundus devoid of pigment. Only the choroidal vessels prevent the sclera from appearing completely white

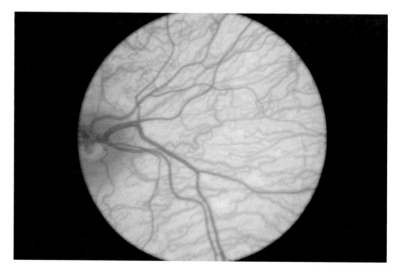

Such eyes do not see well, not only because of absent pigment layer metabolites, but also because the existing retina is overwhelmed by the light presented.

alpha agonists drugs like brimonidine which act on the alpha$_2$ receptors, decreasing the aqueous inflow and increasing the uveo-scleral outflow. They have no cardiac or pulmonary side effects.

antibacterials topical applications customary for ocular infection. Chloramphenicol, framycetin, gentamicin and neomycin have a particularly wide spectrum. Gentamicin and tobramycin are used selectively to deal with *Pseudomonas aeruginosa*. Fusidic acid is of particular use in staphylococcal infections.

amaurosis fugax the 'g' is usually pronounced as a 'j', against all rules of English. It means transient visual loss either of one eye or one field.

amblyopia formal term for a lazy eye. The central vision is diminished or lost in the eye with otherwise no demonstrable physical defect.

angle closure when sudden, is usually known as acute glaucoma. Rarely the block may be chronic and hence without symptoms.

aniridia congenital absence of the iris.

aniseikonia each eye perceives visual perceptions of the same object as different in size. An obstacle to binocular vision.

anisometropia another obstacle to binocular vision. It results from a discrepancy between the refractive needs of each eye. Uncorrected or uncorrectable, it can result in amblyopia (laziness) of the eye with the greater refractive error.

anophthalmos the extremely rare absence of a genuine eyeball.

anterior chamber space bounded in front by the cornea, behind by the iris and filled with aqueous fluid that enters through the pupil and leaves through the trabecular meshwork in the angle.

aphakia absence of the natural lens.

aphasia a synonym for dysphasia: may be receptive or expressive and usually a combination of both. The expressive type is essentially a disorder in language construction but not of comprehension, giving rise to extreme and wholly understandable distress. Receptive dysphasia is a disorder of language analysis. An affected individual can neither appreciate nor act upon instructions. Location of the cause is not always easy but receptive dysphasia incriminates the dominant temporo-parietal lobe. Expressive dysphasia, on the other hand, must incriminate the motor cortex.

aqueous   clear salt solution that fills the anterior chamber and provides a blood substitute for the transparent tissues, cornea, lens and vitreous.

artificial tears   available in liquid or gel preparation, they can be used in the long term management of those eyes where the basal tear flow is drying up.

asteroid hyalitis   star like bodies, suspended in the vitreous, that cause great consternation when they are caught glistening in the light of an ophthalmoscope, which as usual, is vainly in search of something else.

They are not a sign of vitritis and almost never noticed by their owner.

Figure 28.2
Asteroid hyalitis. An undiscovered galaxy to its owner, it is an incidental finding on ophthalmoscopy

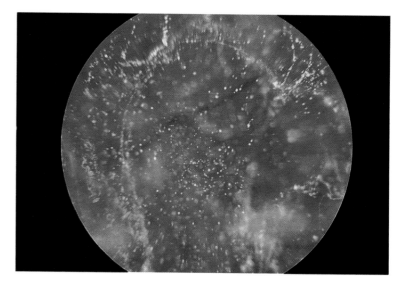

astigmatism   error of refraction which prevents light from coming to a point focus on the retina because focusing mechanisms are not spherical but oval.

atropine sulphate   *see* cycloplegics

beta-blockers   beta-adrenoreceptor-blocking agents are now the sheet anchor in the treatment of raised intraocular pressure. They reduce the inflow and increase the outflow. They may produce deposits on contact lenses to the point where they are mutually exclusive. All beta-blockers slow the heart and may precipitate cardiac failure. Some may cause asthma and the lipid-soluble variety can affect the brain, bringing about hallucinations and disturbance of sleep. Although timolol and carteolol are more effective in absolute reduction of intraocular pressure, there is some evidence that betaxolol preserves the visual field for longer.

binocular vision capacity of the eyes to work together, focusing and fusing images viewed from slightly different angles into one three-dimensional image.

blepharitis inflammation of the skin of the eyelids. There is usually scaling around the lash margin, producing a sort of eyelid dandruff. A destructive ulcerative form is very rare.

buphthalmos now taken as synonymous with infantile glaucoma. The enlarged eyeball with its stretched sclera resembling that of an ox is thought to be the result of raised intraocular pressure in infancy.

Figure 28.3
The large irritable eye of infantile glaucoma

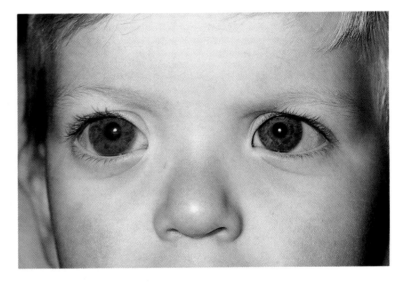

canaliculi drainage ducts for tears in the upper and lower eyelids connecting the lacrimal puncta with the common canaliculus, which itself enters the lacrimal sac.

canthus name given to the angle where the upper lid joins the lower lid.

capsular thickening the posterior capsule, deliberately left behind during extracapsular cataract extraction, may sometimes opacify in the months or years following surgery.

carbonic anhydrase inhibitors the original diuretics, the most celebrated of which is acetazolamide. They reduce aqueous production but in the long term have certain side effects. Acetazolamide has now more even release of the drug than has hitherto been possible. There is some evidence that the systemic malaise previously ascribed to the drug itself has actually been caused by uneven absorption.

carotico-cavernous sinus fistula pulsing proptosis, the rare sequel of traumatic leakage from the carotid artery into the cavernous sinus.

cataract any opacification of the natural lens.

central serous retinopathy an uncommon optic deviation of the macula in non-elderly males, associated with blurring of central vision which usually recovers spontaneously over several weeks. It can effect both eyes at different times and occasionally requires active and not always successful intervention with laser photocoagulation.

chalazion the quiescent end-result of inflammation of one of the tarsal glands.

chloramphenicol most popular topical broad-spectrum antibacterial agent. It retains its efficacy best when stored in a refrigerator. Rate reports of aplastic anaemia through systemic absorption of eye drops cannot be regarded as a serious contraindication to its use.

choroid posterior section of the uveal tract providing the red reflex visible to the ophthalmoscope through the transparent retina.

chloroquine widely used in the management of certain collagen disorders such as systemic lupus erythematosus and rheumatoid arthritis and as a prophylaxis against malaria. White subepithelial corneal deposits have been described in some 30% of patients on long term treatment. Disturbance of the retinal pigment epithelium can result in central loss and constriction of the peripheral fields. Up to 1 g a day in the short term is the accepted safe level, but there is a cumulative effect in the long term.

chorioretinitis (active) the active phase is the first step on the way to a chorioretinal scar. It may arise in the wake of other diseases but is frequently an inflammation in its own right, often without any known cause. The traditional marks of inflammation collect in a white patch in the posterior pole throwing inflammatory debris into the vitreal cavity.

chorioretinitis (healed) the fluffy white patches of active inflammation form into a scar. Destruction of more delicate tissues, like the choroid, the pigment retina and the neuroretina allow the sclera to dominate. White is therefore the first element of the chorioretinal scar. Because there has been an active battle, the one layer that is capable of proliferation will proliferate. Irregular patches of pigment scatter over the white sclera, presiding over the atrophy of everything else.

Figure 28.4
Healed chorioretinitis. All scars, although different in size and location, look the same. Inflammation destroys the choroid and the two retinae, allowing the white sclera to shine through choroidal remnants and fragments of pigment

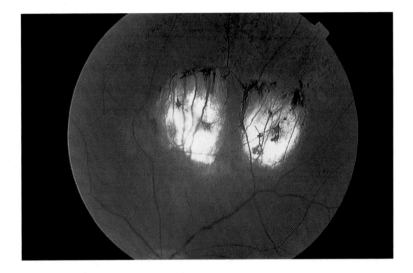

All chorioretinal scars look the same, with white sclera being visible through a broken lacework of chorioretinal remnants, whirls and smudges of black pigment and fibrous tissue in a circumscribed patch, surrounded by normal red reflex. It is perfectly possible to fill out several chapters on the subject of these scars, but it would also be pointless. Whatever their cause, they are all the same.

The positions may be different, with different distribution. The named infections with toxoplasma or toxocara, in solitary circumscribed patches, are of no consequence unless they threaten the macula. Fluffy clouds blur their edges when they are preparing to erupt again.

Laser scars are distributed in a regular pattern in the fundus of a patient who should manage to tell us what has happened.

Cryopexy scars after retinal surgery, eclipse burns and the peppered distribution of syphilitic chorioretinitis somehow continue to slip from one edition to the next without ever being seen today. They all show the common features of a white sclera dominant through a broken choroid with pigment clumps to indicate a past struggle.

ciliary body   middle portion of the uveal tract connecting the iris to the choroid. The natural lens is suspended from the ciliary processes. The ciliary muscle is the muscle of accommodation. The ciliary epithelium, providing the aqueous fluid, is the heart of the eye.

coloboma   persistence of primitive vascular tissue together with failure of fusion of the developing optic vessel results in a congenital cleft of varying dimensions in the lower nasal quadrant. It may range from a slight notch in the eyelid to a complete gap in the uveal tract all the way back to the optic nerve head.

colour vision (and defects)   the eye perceives light between 400 and 700 nm and perceives colour with its colour receptors. Each cone has a maximal perception of red, green or blue. Ocular perception depends on the nature of the ambient light. It is customary to describe colour in terms of hue, brightness and saturation. The hue depends on reflection, radiation or transmission of light of particular wavelengths. Shading is brought about by the addition of black. Brightness is related to light intensity. Saturation indicates the purity of a particular hue. Colour blindness is usually inherited as an X-linked characteristic and apart from exclusion from certain occupations, should not cause any serious visual disturbance.

conjunctiva   wet membrane formed in loose folds between the eyelid and the eyeball. It is like the synovial sac of a ball and socket joint.

convergence   act of pulling the visual axes out of parallel for near vision.

cornea   transparent anterior wall of the eye, continues with the sclera and the anterior limit of the anterior chamber.

corticosteroids   widely used in ophthalmology to suppress inflammation, particularly of idiopathic iritis and that produced by surgery. Also the cause of many complications both short term and long term: they can catastrophically accelerate the corneal destruction in herpes simplex keratitis; they may raise the intraocular pressure in sensitive individuals (steroid responders) and induce posterior subcapsular cataract.

cryocoagulation   the favoured inflammatory insult delivered to the eye during retinal surgery.

crystalline lens   the convex focusing device suspended from the ciliary processes separating the vitreal cavity from the anterior chamber. The term 'crystalline' is going out of fashion.

cycloplegics   drugs that paralyse the ciliary muscle and accommodation, resulting in a dilated pupil and failure to near vision. Atropine is the most famous and long-acting but is now used only in the treatment of iritis. Simple dilatation is brought about by cyclopentolate and, more recently, tropicamide, the action of which wears off in a morning. Adrenaline is not a cycloplegic. It stimulates the dilator pupillae directly.

cylindrical lens   used in the treatment of astigmatism, it focuses in one meridian only.

dacrocystitis   infection that sometimes ends in an abscess of the tear sac.

dark adaptation   the capacity of the retina to increase its sensitivity in response to decreased illumination. It fails in retinitis pigmentosa and other destructive disorders of the peripheral retina, such as pan-retinal photocoagulation.

dioptre   unit by which the strength of lenses is measured.

diplopia   double vision. Monocular implies some opacity. Binocular indicates a paralysis of an extraocular muscle or imbalance of the eyes.

dorzalamide   the topical carbonic anhydrase inhibitor with an effectivity somewhere between timolol and betaxolol.

ectropion   separation between (usually) the lower lid and the eyeball. Hereditary in bloodhounds, the unfortunate result of passing time in the rest of us. In both circumstances the eyes become dry, exposed and inflamed.

endophthalmitis   gross intraocular inflammation, usually the result of infection.

enophthalmos   reverse of proptosis. The eyeball sinks into the orbit, either because of orbital fracture or because of spontaneous shrinkage of the globe itself.

entropion   reverse of ectropion. The eyelid turns inwards, abrading the cornea with the lashes.

enucleation   surgical removal of the eye.

epiphora   another term for watering.

'E' test   testing of visual acuity in those who for one reason or another cannot read.

Excimer laser   a method of sculpting the corneal curvature to reduce myopia and astigmatism.

exenteration   extirpation of the entire contents of the orbit down to the bone, usually for advanced intraorbital malignancy.

exophthalmos   another name for proptosis: the eyeball in advance of where it ought to be.

flashing lights   the demotic term for photopsiae. The retina being light-sensitive will respond to any stimulus in this way. It does not always mean either a retinal break or a retinal detachment. If occurring in one visual field it has a cerebral origin.

floaters   opacities, usually in the vitreous but sometimes in the anterior chamber, recognized by patients in their field of vision. Most floaters appear the same. It is their companions that determine their significance.

fluorescein   sodium fluorescein outlines defects in the corneal epithelium. The sterile strip preparation is favoured for not encouraging the growth of *Pseudomonas pyocyaneus*, an organism that favours only one medium over fluorescein and that being the corneal epithelium itself.

fovea   the absolute centre of the macula where the most exact detail is noted.

fundus   the interior of the eye as seen with the ophthalmoscope.

fusidic acid   broad spectrum antibiotic most effective against staphylococci. Delivered as viscous drops, which do not blur vision whilst remaining active, on a twice-daily basis.

gentamicin   broad spectrum antibiotic in drop or ointment form.

glaucoma   the most precise meaning is an optic neuropathy characterized by particular field defects and disc cupping and usually related to raised intraocular pressure. It also is taken to mean the named disease chronic simple glaucoma. The confusion is compounded by five other meanings: acute glaucoma (angle closure); any rise of intraocular pressure be the cause known or not; any rise of intraocular pressure where the cause is identified (secondary glaucoma); buphthalmos – infantile glaucoma. It would make most sense to reserve the name for the pathological process and describe everything else as a raised intraocular pressure.

guttae   Latin plural of 'gutta' meaning drop. Precedes name of drug prescribed in drop form, e.g. guttae (G) chloramphenicol.

hemianopia   field loss affecting one half of the field of vision of one eye. When both right fields or both left fields are affected we use the term homonymous.

hippus   although the name might suggest some large muscular animal, it refers to small muscular movements in the iris – fine rhythmic minute dilatation and constriction. It is of no consequence.

hordeolum commonly known as a stye. It is indeed much less common than an infected tarsal cyst.

hypermetropia (long sight) error of refraction which forces the eye to focus as for reading when it is seeing in the distance. Even the young eye may have used up all its reading focus when it actually tries to see for near.

intrinsic sympathomimetic activity (ISA) certain compounds both antagonize and stimulate adrenergic receptors. In theory at least they are less likely to cause bradycardia and coldness of the extremities.

Ishihara plates colour test for red–green colour defects. Operated by asking patients to recognize numbers, trace lines and recognize jumbles against a series of multicoloured dots.

keratoconus deformity where the natural dome shape of the cornea gives way to that of a cone.

latanoprost a new drug in the treatment of raised intraocular pressure. A prostaglandin that increases uveo-scleral outflow.

laser acronym from Light Amplification by Stimulated Emission of Radiation. An artificial method of selecting a wavelength of light which may then be directed with great accuracy to any spot within the eye. As the wavelength moves towards the red end of the spectrum its absorption moves deeper through the pigment epithelium into the choroid. Not the treatment of choice for retinal detachment.

Lebers congenital amaurosis total blindness present probably at birth but usually detected later and probably of recessive inheritance.

Lebers optic neuropathy bilateral diminution of central vision to about 6/24 with eventually partial optic atrophy in young males.

limbus margin between the sclera and the cornea. Limbal injection or certain corneal injection is the deep redness indicating one of the three serious red eyes.

macula posterior pole temporal to the optic nerve head centred on the fovea – the acute area of central vision.

macroaneurysm sac-like focal dilatation of retinal arterioles sometimes found in patients with hypertension. Though rare, they tend to occur at the posterior pole and can be a source of vitreal haemorrhage or macular oedema.

microaneurysm sac-like focal pouches that form in retinal capillaries as a classic early sign of background diabetic retinopathy.

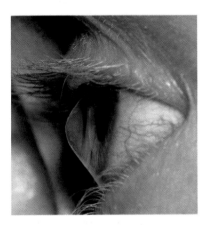

Figure 28.5
Keratoconus. The cornea, like a volcano in shape, can, if thin enough, resemble a volcano in action, expelling the iris like lava through the ruptured cornea

microphthalmos   congenital defect resulting in a tiny and usually useless eyeball.

miotics   drugs which produce constriction of the pupil. They may also drag on the peripheral retina. The only one now used in ophthalmology is pilocarpine.

mydriatics   drugs which cause dilatation of the pupil with or without paralysing the ciliary muscle. Adrenaline or its pro-drug dipivefrin or phenylephrine produce mydriasis by stimulation of the sympathetic nervous system.

myopia   (short sight)   error of refraction in which the eye cannot see in the distance. The distance focus is close to the eye and the near focus closer still.

non-steroidal anti-inflammatory agents   a topical drug which can suppress ocular inflammation as effectively as corticosteroids without raising the pressure, causing cataract or fostering infection has for years been a philosopher's stone for the pharmaceutical chemists. The most recent, diclofenac sodium, would appear to meet all these requirements more impressively than its predecessors.

nystagmus   rapid involuntary movement of the eye at any speed in any direction.

oculentum   Latin singular for ointment: precedes name of drug in ointment form, e.g. oculentum (Oc) chloramphenicol.

one-response organ   each part of the eye tends to have one single response to a whole range of pathological insults.

phakomatoses   a rare collection of lumps scattered throughout the body as well as the eye, and hovering uneasily between the title of genuine tumour and embryonic remnants, their names read like characters from a Lehar operetta: Von Recklinghausen, Von Hippel–Lindau, Bourneville and Sturge–Weber.
   Café au lait spots, skin tumours, intracranial gliomata, angiomatous malformations, sebaceous adenomata and so on will produce local damage and disorder wherever they alight. Fortunately they are as rare as they are untreatable.

pinguecula   a small sessile fatty deposit adjacent to the corneo-scleral limbus which may be mistaken for pterygium.

photocoagulation   technique to produce a chorioretinal scar by the absorption of light and its conversion to heat by the pigment epithelium.

posterior vitreous detachment   a popular explanation for light flashing and floaters when no retinal break can be found. A retina cannot detach until the vitreous has at least liquefied adjacent to a retinal break, probably diagnosed more often than it actually occurs.

presbyopia   refractive state of advancing years when the hardening lens no longer responds to the demands of the ciliary muscle.

preservatives   the chemical integrity of most topical preparations is preserved by other chemicals such as benzalkonium chloride and prolonged treatment with any of them is toxic to the corneal epithelium.

proptosis   eyeball pushed forwards out of the orbit.

pterygium   overgrowth of episcleral and subconjunctival tissues which moves across the cornea, usually from the nasal limbus. Common in desert dwellers, sailors and skiers.

ptosis   drooping of the upper eyelid.

retina   actually splits into the **neuro-retina** and the *pigment retina*. The neuro-retina contains the light-sensitive elements necessary for vision. This layer is potentially separable from the pigment layer. Both layers become adherent at the ora serrata and at the optic nerve head.

retinal detachment   when the neuro-retina separates from the pigment retina usually because of the passage of liquid vitreous through a retinal break.

rheumatoid arthritis   The eye is a small ball and socket joint, a victim to the unexplained disturbance of inflammatory arthritis. The manifestations include episcleritis, a raised red nodule or scleritis – disseminated scleral redness. Deep involvement of the sclera or cornea can result in extreme thinning and sometimes frank perforation.

scotoma   area within the visual field either (a) partially insensitive – **relative**, when a larger object will be seen in better illumination, or (b) totally insensitive – **absolute**, when no object is seen no matter how large or how good the illumination.

Snellen chart   the series of letters used to check the level of distance vision.

Still's disease   juvenile rheumatoid arthritis which gives rise to crippling joint disease and progressive intractable blinding iritis.

strabismus   squint.

sympathetic ophthalmitis   a pan-uveitis involving both eyes following a penetrating injury in one eye.

synechia adhesion of the iris to anything within the anterior chamber.

tobacco alcohol amblyopia heavy consumers of alcohol who reflect on their loss of appetite with tobacco may, over the years, begin to lose their central vision. Failing red/green discrimination and eventual optic atrophy only confirms the suspicion that the history should have already raised.

Cyanide from powerful tobacco overwhelms the enzyme systems that would in normal circumstances have turned it into harmless thiocyanate. This decline of macular function can be halted by parenteral hydroxocobalamine 1000 mg twice weekly.

Tonic pupil (Holmes–Adie) large pupil which responds with maddening slowness both to the presence and absence of light and accommodation. Classically linked to absent deep tendon jerks.

Toxocara (toxocariasis) infection of children who ingest toxocara ova is the reason dogs' fouling streets and parks has become politically incorrect. It should not be forgotten that cats have their own intestinal parasite. The behaviour of both is the same. The larvae die when they reach the retina and produce a violent inflammation within the vitreal cavity producing white exudates, cataracts and possibly anterior chamber inflammation as well.

Toxoplasmosis Toxoplasma gondii is an intracellular protozoan. The clinical appearances clearly depend on where it lands but the infection accounts for almost 30% of all cases of posterior uveal inflammation. Dogs and cats are known to carry these parasites. The inflammation is usually more focal than that of toxocara.

trabeculectomy the favoured surgical procedure to create a passage for aqueous from the anterior chamber to the subconjunctival space.

uveal tract iris, ciliary body and choroid, so named from its resemblance, through a thin sclera, to a black grape.

uveitis one of the synonyms for inflammation of the uveal tract.

viscous drops an ointment which turns into a drop on contact with the eye – sustaining the release of a drug over a prolonged period without blurring the vision.

vitreous the transparent jelly which fills the ocular cavity behind the lens. Like the retina it is adherent at the ora serrata and at the optic nerve head. There is a weaker connection over the macula.

Yag laser (Yttrium Aluminium Garnet) the instrument used to disrupt thickened posterior capsules following cataract surgery. Although miraculously effective in most cases, it can set off shock waves which in turn may produce an intractable retinal detachment in vulnerable eyes.

29

Examinations: how to pass them

The popular cameo of an examination is a confrontation, a duel between some monstrous creation of Roald Dahl and some helpless student whose life of innocent pleasure has left but little time for study. And behind the scenes, nights of frenzy and huge textbooks which defend their contents against a determined attempt to convert them into a last minute imitation of scholarship.

The resultant failure, or scraped pass, then confirms the belief that examinations are just short of armed combat and that they can be passed only by hoodwinking the examiner with a parade of small-print obscurities. In fact, examiners are not so easily taken in and most candidates who fail, do so because they have not grasped the large-print principles.

Any examination can be turned into an easy canter by a little understanding of how it is structured, an understanding of how examiners think and what they are looking for, and by not wasting time studying the same thing in three or four different ways.

Sadly most students give no thought contemplating any of these and rush away in search of medico-babble which they hope will give the impression of fathomless depths of erudition, judgement and wisdom.

How to study
Know your examination; reconnoitre the ground if you must treat it as war. A printed syllabus takes the place of a battle map, giving some indication of the campaign. Talking to successful candidates can be useful; talking to failed candidates is less useful; talking to an examiner will give the view of the other side of the table and need not be regarded as crawling.

The art of study is to recognize what is essential and what is decoration and not to waste time studying the same subject in several different ways in several different books because their fundamental similarity is obscured by slight variations of emphasis and major variations of language.

As an example taken from my own student days, psychiatrists taught us how to diagnose schizophrenia and, during the same term, a police surgeon taught us how to decide if a motorist had consumed more alcohol than was strictly safe. The essence of both was to demonstrate dislocation from reality – in one case, because of psychosis and in the other because of intoxication. The whole of medicine and its related subjects are shot through with many such examples – apparently disconnected yet each capable of description as one set of principles with one set of words.

In the pre-clinical years, each time the instruction manual dissected its way to a new anatomical region – from the axilla to the hand, from the abdomen to the feet – it uncovered peripheral nerves snaking between the muscles. Each time one was named, so was its inevitable spray of branches to skin, follicles, blood vessels and so on and students then had to learn several times something that required learning only once.

These branches are the same, whether they sprout from the ulnar nerve or the sciatic nerve and the major portion of a distinguished answer in regional anatomy can be constructed from them before any mention has to be made of where they actually are.

If picking up the thread that links essentials is the first step, then the second is to form an opinion about them – all of them; this fixes them in the mind as golden nuggets of genuine knowledge, the glitter of which sheds light on any dark gaps uncovered in between them by hard questioning.

This habit of reasoning around fundamentals, polished in practice, hardens into a gleaming surface that will not crack in the white heat of an examination.

The study of all clinical subjects can be as ordered as the study of anatomy. Although the details may change we need frameworks which are unchanging, and indeed which belong to all branches of medicine. Any clinical subject can be studied and answered on the basis of four cardinal elements:

- pathology
- essential symptoms
- essential signs
- essential management.

- We know that the eye is an organ of limited response. We also know that, should the condition in question produce some remote complication, there is a fair chance that it will involve the aqueous dynamics and the intraocular pressure. It cannot be difficult to find parallels between this and any other branch of medicine we care to mention.

- There are but five essential symptoms and we can work out from the processes of pathology which of these symptoms might be triggered and why.
- The essential signs do not change from condition to condition although decades of ophthalmic teaching would have us believe that they do.
- Essential management is the same, no matter what part of the body is involved. We have to:

(a) diagnose and find the cause
(b) eliminate the cause if we can
(c) deal with the effects of the cause (complications)
(d) relieve pain
(e) restore function.

All this can be attempted by *medical* means or *surgical* means – first of all in the *short term* and secondly in the *long term*.

The preceding framework must be in position before the examination, in the subconscious mind at the brain-stem level, releasing the conscious mind to observe, reason and respond at speed in the certainty that nothing has been missed.

WRITTEN PAPERS

The prime aim in any examination is to persuade the examiners that you have an ordered mind, that you grasp your subject and that you do not pad out your answers with question-begging, special pleading and needless repetition.

Even less convincing is the answer, for which an hour was allowed, scribbled over half a page, with the postscript 'time' – somehow meant to suggest a brain so teeming with information that an hour was not long enough to allow the candidate to decide what should be left out.

The written examination is the ideal opportunity to notch up extra marks at leisure, because there is no face-to-face contact with an examiner whom the candidate might perceive as awesome.

The injunction not to study twice what needs to be studied only once applies equally to the construction of written answers. Every statement of consequence should be defended. An examiner will not be impressed by an inventory of capital words, stressing that the management of some disorder or another is important because it is serious, because it is vital, because it is critical. These are simply repetitions of something not yet proven.

The treatment of iritis is not 'steroids, four times a day'. This level of answer simply will not do. We have to define the problem – inflammation of the iris, which if untreated may lead on to:

- a secondary rise of pressure
- adhesions between the iris and the lens
- destruction of the eye
- cataract
- spontaneous resolution.

The treatment, slotting into its place in the framework of management in general is then the suppression of that inflammation with topical corticosteroids because, if it is not suppressed, then these possible complications might follow. That said, there is then no need to keep reminding the examiner that the inflammation has to be suppressed.

We should now be in a position to construct an answer on, say, herpes zoster ophthalmicus – the aetiology, pathology, clinical features, complications and management. This may sound alarming, but it is absolutely founded on simple principles and might read as follows:

ANSWER

Space demands that this be constructed in note form. However, in the examination, a major answer should be constructed as an essay, which of course implies the use of sentences and some attempt at literary composition.

The **diagnosis** is made from the classical distribution of the vesicles.

Management

Problems
- Dermatitis. Infection of the broken vesicles. Scar formation. Late intractable pain.
- Conjunctivitis. Pain. Secondary infection.
- Keratitis.
  Acute. Loss of vision due to superficial punctate keratitis.
  Chronic. Corneal scars if the active lesions penetrate Bowman's membrane.
  Cornea vulnerable because of virus-induced anaesthesia.
- Iritis.
  Acute. Pain. Loss of vision. Floaters.
  Chronic. Adhesions. Iris to the lens. Secondary glaucoma.
  Damage to the trabecular meshwork. Secondary rise in pressure, cataract.

Treatment

- *Dermatitis*

  Short term: The aim is to kill the virus and to allow bacteria-free healing with minimal scar formation.

  Acyclovir skin cream five times daily deals with the first problem. Thereafter an application which combines an antibiotic with corticosteroid may achieve both these aims to some degree. Their dosage will depend on the severity of the condition.

  Long term: The pain of shingles is devastating and long term analgesics and emotional support may still not be enough to prevent thoughts of suicide.

- *Conjunctivitis*

  The aim is to prevent secondary infection from spreading to the cornea.

  The application of topical antibiotics in a dose related to the severity usually achieves the above aims.

- *The cornea*

  Short term: Breach of corneal epithelium. The aim is to persuade the epithelium to heal. This is one condition where the danger of topical corticosteroids in the presence of a broken corneal epithelium is outweighed by their benefit in suppressing inflammation. But sometimes circumstances have to be created to allow the cornea to heal in its own time.

  Closure of the eyelids with adhesive tape is ideal, but may not be easy because the broken skin on the eyelids might prevent the tape from sticking, whilst severe iritis requires constant topical treatment.

  Frequent application of artificial tears goes some way to making the cornea feel that the eyelids are closed, which is its ideal state, even in health.

  Long term: An anaesthetic cornea is a vulnerable cornea, and years after the acute attack this may lead to recurrent breakdown of the corneal epithelium.

  Tape closure is by far the best way to give the cornea the circumstances it likes best.

  When the cornea has recovered, it may be kept that way by closing the eyelids from time to time (perhaps one weekend out of three) on a regular basis. There is no precise time scale.

- *Iritis*

  The aim is to suppress inflammation and prevent complications in the acute phase.

  Complications and restoration of function dominate the management of the chronic phase.

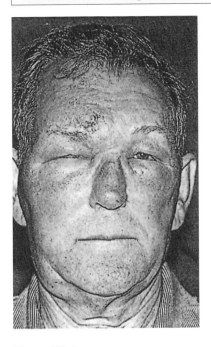

Figure 29.1
Herpes zoster ophthalmicus –
ophthalmic shingles due to infection
along the first division of the
trigeminal nerve. With the advent of
acyclovir, the full-blown florid
picture is becoming a rarity

Short term:
Topical corticosteroids – the dose is related to the severity of the inflammation.

Mydriatics – if the pupil shows signs of adhering to the lens, then dilating it will make the development of adhesions less likely to be complete.

If the intraocular pressure be raised, then it must be brought down.

Acetazolamide reduces the production of aqueous. However, it also produces systemic effects in the form of increased diuresis, finger tingling, kidney stones, metabolic acidosis and possibly even mental upset.

Topical beta-blockers – these drugs also reduce the production of aqueous, but with fewer side effects in most patients. However, they can delay the healing of corneal epithelium, and indeed may cause an intact epithelium to break down.

Long term:
The intraocular pressure may remain permanently raised and will therefore require long-term treatment, possibly with beta-blockers or other anti-glaucoma drugs, or even drainage surgery. This is the age of chronic simple glaucoma and we must be sure that the condition we are dealing with really is secondary.

Cataract: There should be no particular complication in the removal of cataract. It is always best to restore the lost focus with an intraocular lens, but if there are problems in controlling intraocular pressure before surgery, these may be worse after surgery, and may indeed require further surgery to control them.

Treatment before disease is established. The best management of all would be to abort all complications before they come into being. This can sometimes be achieved by systemic acyclovir if we can catch the disease in its prodromal phase.

The flaw in this approach is that we must catch the condition almost before we know what it is. People tend to put up with pain in the forehead; it is only the appearance of vesicles and worse that persuade them to seek attention.

Acyclovir tablets are expensive. The dosage is four times the standard – 800 mg five times daily for 7 days. But treating the complications in their full flower is probably more expensive still, not to mention the price in continued misery.

The pedestrian simplicity of this answer must come as a disappointment to all those who are seeking the passport to that rarified wonderland – that Arcania where the most unlikely conditions are diagnosed by guesswork, then confirmed by the most uncommon investigations and then treated by the most radical stratagems imaginable – clearly a land where canaries dare and where no sparrows fly.

ORAL EXAMINATIONS

Ideally these meetings should be conducted as conversations between equals, and if they are not, the fault almost invariably lies with the candidate.

The quality of response is measured by order, grasp of fundamentals and the very sensible realization that the examiner is looking for large-print principles and not a word-for-word repetition of page 2000 from whatever textbook happens to be the fashion of the year.

Any human meeting is an interplay of personality quirks, frailties and deeply held convictions. It is not the examiners alone who have a monopoly of personality flaws. At least, examination bodies try to root them out on their side of the table. However, they have no power to do the same thing for the candidates. The total elimination of human oddities would be impossible because indeed they are the warp and weft of life. In any case, after the examination – and there is life after the examination – successful candidates will encounter eccentricities far worse than anything conjured up at a Royal College of this or that.

CANDIDATES

Apart from frank ignorance, which may be the result of opening too many rather than too few textbooks, candidates regularly fail examinations for the following reasons:

- They have no ordered framework for study.
- They have formed no opinions of their own.
- They waste time discovering the pet subjects of local examiners hoping to greet each with an inventory of their favourite beliefs. That they may have been misinformed or that it was all worthless information anyway never seems to put an end to this traffic in misguided faith.
- Their brains are top-heavy with small-print minutiae at the expense of large-print essentials.
- They fancy that they and the examiner have memorized the same book and that success must come mechanically if they can only identify which page the examiner has in mind, whereupon the pair of them can sit back to enjoy a shared memory.

Examiners do not memorize textbooks and they certainly do not read them up for the examination. Candidates, particularly those for whom English is not their native tongue, would spare themselves much unhappiness if they grasped this fact now, because if they do not, they will find themselves not only not enjoying a shared memory but perhaps being told that although the memory may be right, the content is wrong.

Most candidates believe that the examiner will be impressed if they can discharge all their detailed knowledge immediately, preferably in one sentence. Even if the torrent of information were intelligible it leaves the candidate nothing to decorate bare principles with later. No examiner will ever quibble with a general statement first. In fact they invariably prefer answers given that way.

So a question on the principles of applanation tonometry should not release an instant flood of detail about the formula for the area of a circle, the constituents of the ideal fluorescein anaesthetic mixture, a disquisition on surface tension and on the dangers of infection.

The opening statement must surely be that applanation tonometry is a way of measuring intraocular pressure; that a flat surface is applied to a curved surface at an increasing pressure. When the area of contact flattens, the pressure within equals the pressure without. That may well be enough. If details are asked then the questions will guide the candidate into which details are needed.

A good working rule is that we should always ask ourselves first, is there some prefatory statement that should have been made before the statement that is actually being made – some peg of first principles on which to hang later details?

Someone is bound to be asked about Horner's syndrome, and is equally likely to release a breathless list of causes, involving fractures of the cervical vertebra, tabes dorsalis, syringomyelia, apical tuberculosis and so on. The syndrome may indeed be caused by all of these things but that does not give any clue to the examiner that this is not just simply a list memorized from a huge textbook.

We could be tempted to say that Horner's syndrome is caused by paralysis of the cervical sympathetic nervous system, but it is possible that we should take one step further back still and describe it as an affection of one eye characterized by ptosis and miosis – because that is the first thing we see. The next statement could implicate the cervical sympathetic and thereafter, if asked, the more common causes could be considered.

The concept of syndromes is not encouraged in this book but medicine would not be medicine without a bit of tradition. The syndromes of tradition should at least form familiar patterns, but what should be the response to questions about a 30-year-old with sudden onset of horizontal diplopia?

The answer is not a salvo of pathology from demyelination to an intracranial aneurysm – though one of them may
be to blame. We must first define the problem and break it
up into categories. Is the diplopia monocular or binocular?
If binocular, is it a latent squint breaking down, a frank
paralysis of an extraocular muscle, or is the latter
masquerading as the former? Each category is then open for
discussion and wise candidates can direct that discussion to
where they feel most comfortable.

The greatest source of disquiet to an examiner is the candidate who does not answer the question but sits paralysed in
a long and terrible silence. This absence of speech can be
quite as destructive as the gush of detail. The most likely
cause is an instinctive assumption that the answer must be
in detail, and no detail comes to mind. The answer, dare we
repeat it again, should be in principle and no candidate
should approach an examination bereft of basic principles.

For those whose mother tongue is not English, it is as
well to learn several ways of phrasing the same idea well in
advance of the examination. It makes things needlessly difficult if, in addition to the subject under scrutiny, the connecting phrases have to be continually translated into an
unfamiliar tongue.

These phrases should be constructed for multiple use,
ready to be deployed for strange subjects, unexpected
subjects and examiners who appear to be beyond pleasing.
If the linguistic translations are prepared in advance, then
the conscious mind is free for the imaginative leaps necessary to keep the oral examination ticking along.

We have also to recognize that candidates meet not only
examiners, they also meet other candidates who all appear
to have been asked terribly clever questions to which they
knew all the terribly clever answers on matters unfamiliar
to everyone else. The rule is to note that, at the end of the
examination, those with the loudest mouths and the clever-
est answers are almost invariably absent from the list when
the successful candidates are posted.

Hopeful examinees often add to their own sense of
anguish with last-minute study. One such has been observed
reading Gray's anatomy whilst attempting to deal with last-
minute spasms of the bladder. Whatever else he passed, it
was not the anatomy examination, although some allowance
should have been made for manual and cerebral dexterity.

EXAMINERS

Examiners do not all come out of the same box. The ideal
examiner will try to put candidates at their ease and ask

one or two personal questions that moisten the tongue and allow it to separate from the palate. Not every examiner, however, is ideal and we have all come across exceptions from time to time. It is important to recognize that, apart from the very odd exception, most examiners think that they are good examiners and are certain that they are motivated by the highest principles. We are all victims of our own self-perception but, if candidates are going to be courtiers, they have to remember that all kings are more or less beautiful. As candidates, therefore, we have to recognize that examiners are in the driving seat and that nothing is to be gained by impertinence, arrogance or dishonesty.

The furrowed brow

Such displays of anguish may have nothing to do with our answers but with the examiner's concern that justice be done. But when every answer is met with a grimace worse than the one before, we might feel in the circumstances that it is we who are responsible. It could well be reasonable then to try to find out if we are disturbing the examiner in some way – asking if the answer was the sort of response that was wanted.

The single answer

Not infrequently a question may be asked with a single answer in mind when there may well be ten other answers, all equally correct. We have all been through it: working our way through an inventory of replies whilst the examiner keeps shaking the head and saying 'But is there not something else?'

If we appear to be getting nowhere near the magic answer and our confidence is collapsing, the way out is to persuade the examiner to recognize that the other answers were all relevant. A straight question as to their relevance might be the simplest stratagem.

A variation on the single answer

This might appear at first to be another version of the last example but it is not. Sometimes examiners might ask candidates to perform a small manoeuvre like tying a surgical knot. Although the term surgical knot is used glibly and frequently, there is no such thing as a surgical knot. The candidate may well realize this and not quite know how to respond when a piece of string is placed on the table.

In these circumstances we take refuge again in first principles. We might answer that knots in surgery (note the use of the words 'surgery' and 'knot' but with the order reversed) will vary in different circumstances and with different suture materials.

The essence of a knot is that it should fulfil its purpose. It should be unobtrusive; it should not slip. The 'sliding granny knot' of retinal surgery would not be suitable for a corneal graft because the surgical needs and the material are different.

That said, there is then no reason why the candidate cannot then tie whatever knot the examiner requests.

The angry examiner

Anger is unforgivable but it does happen from time to time at the end of a long trying day of orals, and it may be brought on by a candidate apparently dodging the issue or avoiding the point or not answering the question asked or simply sitting in silence.

Obviously it is in our interests to understand why the examiner has become irate, if we can and if we have enough conscious mind available to deal with the added pressure. It is at this point that the wisdom of prepared phrases becomes evident.

The first essential is to keep cool, which means counting to three, breathing deeply the while and not bursting into tears. This might well have worked with Napoleon, whom tears generally reduced to impatient blotting paper, but the average male examiner would simply wait for the storm to pass and the average female examiner would probably not wait at all.

Should the anger become intolerable, then it is perfectly reasonable to ask the examiner what we have done to produce such rage – and the phrases we use must of course be tried out and practised before venturing them in the white heat of an examination.

It is helpful sometimes to remind the examiner that we have had a teacher possibly not unlike the person in front of us at the moment and that our whole approach has been taught to us by someone and not just acquired unaided from a textbook.

Expected answer wrong

It has not been unknown for candidates to be asked their opinion of light flashing. We all know that light flashing can have a basis in the retina or in the optic pathways – as far back as the cerebral cortex. If the examiner were to interrupt an answer explaining all this by saying 'no' and that light flashing was caused by retinal detachment, then it is absolutely critical to stick to our point without causing offence.

We might say that we understood that light flashing was due to traction on the retina and that when the retina had torn the light flashing stopped. We might then ask the examiner 'is this not the case?'. If we can then persuade the examiner to join in the discussion, that in fact it might be so, then we have brought things back to the level of discussion and not the realm of machine-gun answering.

When I was a lad

Time catches up with all of us and examiners who have always perceived themselves as young and forward-looking may not have realized that they have become old and backward looking. 'When I was a lad' is a coded message favouring an old technique that may indeed no longer be in use.

Clearly, to say that something is out of date is not wise, particularly if the examiner has fond memories of it. It would, however, be perfectly acceptable to emphasize that our teachers have told us something quite different because of some perfectly valid reason. If this answer can be given in a way that implies that the only real difference is youth and inexperience, then there can be no reason for the examiner to take umbrage.

Examiner with a story

A candidate was once told by the examiner, 'I was at my golf club last night and I woke up blind. What do you think might be wrong?'

It would be easy to imagine ourselves adrift in the quicksands of unreality, expected to provide a diagnosis on half a story and no signs. Most candidates who come to grief do so because they believe that this is the question.

It is not the question. We are being asked not to make a diagnosis immediately but to explain how we would arrive at our diagnosis.

Henry Longhurst used to say that putting was easy once emotion was removed from it. The same goes for the examination. All we need do is reason as we would in our own clinic, except this time in front of an audience. The diagnostic wheels should by now be revolving around:

- possible causation
- symptoms that might belong to the different causes
- signs that would indicate one or other of the likely causes.

Pathology

Conceivable causes of visual loss in a middle-aged man – presumably reasonably fit. If the examiner is portly and florid and breathing with difficulty, that might add a cause or two to our list but of course diplomacy will dictate how far these additions should be put into words.

Symptoms

We must never say 'I would take a good history'. What other history would we take? What we have to say is that we would want to know from the history what the patient meant by blindness. We would have to edit the history and ask questions directed towards whichever of the possible causes we have in mind. Is there total loss of light perception? If not, how much is left? Has it ever happened before? Had anything been consumed in large quantities? – after all it was a golf club and not a church social.

The seven signs

By this time we should, on automatic pilot, have arrived at the conclusion that the reason for bilateral visual reduction to the level of light perception is most likely to be found somewhere in the optic nerves. If the golf club were an essential part of the story and not merely interpolated to add verisimilitude, then the most likely explanation would be a job lot of methanol passed off to the club as whisky.

But suppose the examiner is looking for the single answer of Eales disease, doubtless parrying every correct answer with 'and what else?'

This means the story was a genuine episode and not a fictional tale concocted for the examination. It has to be conceded that bilateral vitreal haemorrhage would not be the first on the list of conditions to explain bilateral blindness. It would therefore be absolutely acceptable to defend a diagnosis of bilateral optic neuritis with edited abstracts from the essential symptoms and from the essential signs.

The message here is loud and clear. It does not always matter if we come to the wrong conclusion, provided we come to it in the right way.

Experience

Occasionally, in a surgical oral, the examiner, in the face of some stumbling answer, might ask if the candidate has done this or that operation before. The answer may well be 'no', but that does not imply that the candidate must fail. The operation may be one that is not practised by every ophthalmologist but by those with a subspecialty.

The response must therefore be not just simply 'no', but 'no' and why. We might say that, where we have trained, this has been considered as a subspecialty operation to be done by an expert only. Thereafter, however, we should then be prepared to go on and discuss the technique. In other words we have not just delivered an unvarnished 'no'. By qualifying it, we have in fact turned our practical inexperience into the positive feature which in fact it is.

CLINICAL EXAMINATIONS

The clinical section of the examination proper is merely an extension of the golfer with the visual handicap and in no way parallels a normal out-patient clinic – but then that is the way of clinical examinations. It is a measure of our skill as a candidate to turn these artificial anomalies of the examination into something that we do every day.

We will almost invariably be asked to do the one thing that this book emphasizes that we should not do – namely to look at a fundus and make a decision without any information from the essential symptoms or the seven signs. We can appear the thoughtful clinicians we really are by recognizing what aspects of real life are missing and by arriving at our diagnosis by the landmarks described above.

Coming to a sensible clinical conclusion face-to-face, be it from a fundal appearance or from a story, calls above all things for a clear, ordered technique, which is as follows:

The eye, dare we repeat it, is an organ or limited response. We must regard each of these responses as a terminus to which lines run from different pathological starting points. Along these lines stops can be made at the essential symptoms and the seven signs. Which of the symptoms and signs we stop at will be determined by the starting point and the terminus. Stopping at them all would clearly take a long time, would certainly irritate the examiner and might end up arriving at the wrong terminus anyway. The secret, as ever, is to edit.

Presented with a terminus (a fundal appearance) we can edit our way back to a starting point. Presented with a starting point we can edit our way down to a terminus.

When it comes to management, we have to remember that **there is no one answer in clinical medicine.**

Clinical responses are complexes of the perceived pathology, the particular needs of the particular patient, the particular views of a clinician, together with experience, past thinking and current thinking on the subject. The examiner doesn't want us to agree for the sake of agreement. What they want to know are our views on the matter, particularly in relation to our experience and why we would undertake such an approach. They want to know, in other words, if we are safe.

If we are left, then, with a fundal appearance, we should always remember that looking at the fundus, particularly with the direct ophthalmoscope, all that will come into view (if anything, indeed) will be the disc, the macula and the vessels. We should form an opinion on these and store that opinion. We should then see if there is any other feature that springs out and, when being asked about it, describe it as the dominant feature. If the examiner then asks 'What about the disc, the macula, the vessels?' then the reflex assimilation of their appearance would be there ready to describe.

It is vital to remember that the management of anything anywhere is to:

- find the cause if we can
- eliminate the causes if we can
- deal with the complications
- relieve pain
- restore function.

Each of these will be weighted differently:

— from medical to surgical
— from short term to long term
— from patient to patient
— from circumstance to circumstance.

But the foundation of successful management is first to define what has to be managed. A binocular grandfather and a monocular boy may both have identical cataracts – but they cannot have identical indications for intervention.

That, then, is the secret of studying, sitting, passing and possibly even enjoying examinations. Although it may not appear obvious, the examiner is not looking to fail but to pass a candidate. It is a great sense of relief and indeed a pleasure when the candidate turns the examination into a discussion between equals. If candidates would only grasp this fact, and exchange a shaky knowledge of small print for a secure knowledge of large print, then there would be fewer drawn and anxious faces on examination day on either side of the table.

Epilogue

The constant theme of this book is the recognition of a safe eye – one that will not go blind because we have missed the things that people do not complain about:

- creeping field loss
- shallow anterior chamber
- raised intraocular pressure.

Such safety can be recognized by going through the ophthalmic ritual of seven markers using the ophthalmoscope only at the end to confirm what we expect to find. In essence this is observation along a subconscious framework, leaving the conscious mind free to speculate on what has been discovered.

A detective, famous for his deerstalker, Stradivarius and curved pipe, made his name synonymous with this technique. He believed there was all the difference in the world between simply looking and looking within a framework which he called observation. His findings were then a product of observation and reason, and by the systematic elimination of whatever could not be possible. His creator, Arthur Conan Doyle, based his character on Joseph Bell, a former president of the Royal College of Surgeons of Edinburgh, whose uncanny deductions from observations of apparently nothing were legendary. Much more significant from our point of view was that Conan Doyle, a doctor, specialized in diseases of the eye.

Index